Getting Out

My Story Plus The Exercises And
Experience I Learned That Can Help You
Get Out From The Wheelchair

GREG SIOFER

Thank You's

There are numerous people who helped along my journey that I would like to thank, but I will stick with the people closest to my heart.

Firstly, I would like to thank God for sticking by me, along with my loving parents, Tadeusz and Urszula Siofer; we have gone through an exceedingly difficult time together. I would especially like to thank my mom for the extremely strong, emotional help I received in Poland.

I would like to thank Dr. D. Milko and his wife Dr. M. Milko, for the numerous physical therapy techniques they taught me.

I would like to thank Dr. Oczkowski, for my neurology care.

Dr. Deveram, for his excellent eye care.

Magdi Boctor, for his support.

Dr. R. DeViller, for saving my life.

Piotr Kaszczuk, for his support.

Patty Barnum, for her support.

Artur and Leszek Lasinski, along with Sylwia Bartnik, Robert Lasinski, and Jola Lasinska, for their friendship and support.

Tadeusz Lasinski and Danuta Lasinska, for their support.

Tadeusz and Alicja Maziarz, for their support.

Paweł and Basia Stołek, for letting us stay with them in Poland and for their support.

Marlena, Luiza and Monika Stołek, for our childhood life refresh and support.

Stefanie Biggar, for our friendship and for the treadmill.

Ursula Köster Páez and her loving family, for helping a stranger.

I would also like to thank my former neighbors, Jim Sawadski and his wife Dawna Sawadski, for their support, prayers, and for the trike. My super former co-workers, Vladamir Spehar and Connie DeChaves, and my former boss, Bonnie Feeney, and her husband, Jim Feeney. And of course, my lovely daughter, Isabella Siofer, for her motivational push and book support.

Things would have turned out differently if I had not had these people by my side. You will meet people on your journey that will help you, and some that will not.

Surround yourself with positive energy, meaning people that want to see you succeed, and get rid of that negative energy. You do not need negative emotions; they will only slow you down.

Dear Reader,

Writing this book has been more emotional than I originally thought it would be. Bringing back my past experiences was extremely difficult; I had to pause numerous times, sometimes only resuming after a few weeks. Even now when I talk about this, I become very emotional, but I know it had to be done so you do not have to go through the same difficulty as I have.

A lot has happened, but I managed to focus on the task ahead and try to recover what walking used to feel like. My greatest motivation was being able to build a snowman with my daughter. Motivation is something you will need to succeed, so find something that motivates you and focus on it.

I wanted to write my story about the difficult time after my procedure, what has happened, and the answers I have received along the way. Throughout my struggle, I always asked people how long it would take until I would recover. There was no book on this subject until now; plus, I always received answers that made no sense. If you are wondering how long your recovery will take, I will answer your question, but the answer might surprise you.

Everyone's recovery time is different depending on the injury they sustained. What may take someone else one year may take you five years; the part of the brain that has been damaged from your stroke, accident, or surgery needs time to relearn. The younger you are, the quicker your recovery will be. Take me as an example: my surgery was in 2008 (aged 27), and I am still not fully recovered.

There are a lot of techniques that can greatly improve your recovery time. One good example is repeating a movement you can no longer do due to the injury that you sustained. If you are not able to write, you practice until you can. Start with making lines, circles, letters, then finally try to make words.

If you are not walking, you practice until you can walk. Think of making small progress before you do any big exercises. You will have muscle weakness after your unfortunate accident; remember you will relearn your movements slower than a young kid learning to walk. So, do not be discouraged by the slow progress you are making. Think of something that can push you.

We often do not appreciate things until we lose them. I know that for myself; I never wondered how I was able to walk, write or throw—I just did, and the question never popped in my mind until I could not do these things. Only then did I look for answers.

You learn the basics at an incredibly young age, so do not expect to relearn everything quickly. If you repeat the movement a lot (and I mean a lot), until that movement becomes automatic, you will not have to think about it; you will just do it. This goes for everything—as of right now, any movement you make is conscious. In a sense, you are retraining the muscles that are required to accomplish your task. I will be focusing on walking, but the same idea goes for other things that you are missing.

I know this is not the answer you were looking for. I know you were expecting an answer with a certain time, but unfortunately, this is not the case and it sucks.

I hope that you can somewhat relate to my story and that the exercises are useful to you. There are a lot of variations on my exercises; however, if you are starting from zero, this will be an excellent book that can provide guidance for your recovery.

Depending on your situation, please be careful and consult with your doctor before proceeding with any exercises.

I hope this book is extremely useful for you; I know it would have been for me after my surgery.

Regards,

Greg Siofer
www.iwillbewalking.com

CONTENTS

Thank You's...iii

Dear Reader, ... v

Chapter 1: The Beginning of My Journey 1

Chapter 2: Doctors Know it All, Right? 5

    The CD 7

    The Failed Eye Cure Attempt... 8

    Getting Contacts.. 9

Chapter 3: Hospital Stay 13

    Time for a Second Opinion 14

Chapter 4: Fed Up 17

Chapter 5: Healer Is a Joke.. 23

    Decision Made.. 25

Chapter 6: First Surgery 27

    Confused About Second Surgery... 28

Chapter 7: Recovery.. 31

    Head Lift 33

Chapter 8: The Outside World 35

    Saliva 38

Chapter 9: Going to Hamilton General Hospital 39

    Throat Hole for Safety 40

    Right Eye Check 41

    Hallway in the Hospital? 41

Chapter 10: Pee I Think... 43

    The Stroll to Start Recovery 44

    3rd Surgery.. 48

Chapter 11: New Room, Strange Dreams..................................51
    Rape Dreams, Are They? 52
    Hand/PT Development 53
Chapter 12: Fit Test to Leave..57
Chapter 13: St. Peter's Hospital, About Time 61
    Food to Fatten Me Up 62
    Roommate 63
    Teaching Me to Eat..63
    First PT..64
    Feeding Practice 65
    Physical Therapy Again 66
    Isabella's First Visit 67
    Trying Coffee When not Allowed 67
Chapter 14: Speech Therapy 71
    PT Continued...74
    Testing My Touch Response.....................................74
    Refusing the Medicine 75
    Stomach Tube Removal..76
Chapter 15: Going Home 79
    Trying Electric Stimulation 80
    An Embarrassing Moment 80
    Diaper Removal Finally..81
    Weekends at Home..81
    Chess With Dad 82
    Out of St. Peter's Hospital and Extremely Excited......82
    Planning a Trip for Adult Stem Cells......................83
Chapter 16: Unexpected Help.......................................85
    Thank You 86
    Hotel in Germany..86
    The Treatment in Germany: Adult Stem Cells 86
    Flight to Poland 88
    Reaching Poland 89
    Cousin Surprise..91
Chapter 17: Physical Therapy in Poland........................93
    Right Eye in Trouble 95
Chapter 18: Separation via MSN Messenger Chat, Really?.............99

Visiting Mom's Place 100
Returning to Canada From Poland 101
Acupuncture Hype Crushed 104
A Friend 105
BrainPort on Trial 105
Chapter 19: Back to Hamilton General 107
Trying Pool PT in the Hospital 107
Surprise Treadmill for Training 109
Isabella's First Communion — I Thought We Were Adults? 110
Strange Experience Still Brings Confusion 111
Facial Nerve Surgery 112
Chapter 20: An Injury and a Surprise 115
Trike Surprise From My Neighbors 117
Shopping Cart From the Grocery Store 118
Moving to My Parents' New Place 120
Surprising Nerve Pinch 121
Finally Made it Happen 123
Isabella 125
Training 127
FAQ 203
Who is Greg Siofer? 205
Request 207

CHAPTER 1

The Beginning of My Journey

Passing cars and seeing stars out the window, the cool night air blew in through the open windows as I hurried home. My wife (at the time) and I had some friends that were getting married soon, and we had invited them over for supper. I had not even had time to get the tortilla chips for the recipe we were planning to make. Hopefully, our friends would arrive late; maybe the traffic out of Toronto would slow them down.

I parked at the house and dashed straight into the kitchen. As I put the chicken and potatoes into the oven, my wife asked about the tortilla chips for the snack. Pretending I had not heard the question, I showed her the red wine I'd grabbed on the way home.

Just then, the doorbell rang. "They're here," I said to her. The table was set with plates, utensils, and wine glasses, and everything seemed ready for us to sit down. Our friends, Lizbeth and Tucker, came in and we all approached the table.

As our friends sat down, my wife went to the kitchen to put the final touches on the food, and I poured the wine to keep them occupied. I took a seat and said cheers and we began to drink from our glasses. Although it was only around 200 mL, and not a strong wine, I noticed that I was already starting to slur my words and get very fidgety as if I had been consuming hard liquor. Confused but not wanting to cause a scene, I pointedly ignored this strange behavior.

When we'd finished our wine, I apologized that we were missing the tortilla chips and offered to walk ten minutes to the convenience store to pick some up, but we decided to go after supper.

My wife and I left the table and went to the kitchen to check on the chicken and potatoes. The chicken was looking brown and juicy so we took it out of the oven and placed it on the counter, and the potatoes were perfectly crispy. We served Tucker and Lizbeth, and I was happy to see how well we had done even though I had been rushing to get things done in time.

With supper over, we walked down the road to the convenience store, glancing up at the stars and just talking about our future. We looked at the other nice houses in our neighborhood, seeing how people lived.

On the way back, I was a bit shaky and flimsy. Again, it felt like I had been drinking quite heavily earlier, which was not the case. I wondered what the heck was happening, but again I stayed silent and ignored whatever was going on, proceeding toward our house and admiring the multi-colored leaves of the trees along our gently curving path. Looking at the sky full of stars, the moon shining bright, and no clouds in sight, helped keep my mind off my body's sudden strangeness.

Back at the house, everything was lit up as if someone was home. We enjoyed a few of the beers that I always kept in the fridge in case of company, then made the snack with the tortilla chips, which turned out to be brownish and crunchy. We had a super time just mumbling about nothing of importance. Our friends spent that night at our place since they were in no shape to be driving—which can happen when you are having a good time and lose count of how much you've had to drink.

I woke up to the sun streaming into my window and proceeded to the washroom, still wobbly. I stared at my face in the mirror and splashed it with cold water, thinking my present unsteadiness would soon go away. But then I looked closer at my eyes and could see that my pupils appeared different than normal, that the black circles in the middle of my eyes were colossal, as if I had been drinking heavily.

Walking unsteadily back to my room, I got dressed and informed my wife that something was off with me, that the unsteadiness had not gone away since yesterday. Still not thinking too much of it, we both headed to the kitchen, where empty bottles sat on the floor and dirty plates were piled on the table.

When Tucker showed up in the kitchen, we decided to drive five minutes to get coffee and bagels. Getting there was a little strange. I got into his sporty car and we immediately blasted the radio. As we pulled out of the driveway, my head began to spin, but I would not let anything divert my attention from the task of getting something to eat. Even as my body hair began to stand up and droplets of sweat appeared on my forehead, I kept pretending everything was okay so as not to cause a scene. At the drive-through, we placed our order of coffee, bagels, and donuts. I was eating my donut when Tucker suddenly pumped the brakes, making the filling of my donut squirt onto my shirt. Then just as quickly he pressed the gas, causing my heart to crash inside my chest. My face was red, and my eyes were wide open. Finally, he released the gas pedal, but I could see lights in the rearview mirror. We double-checked and yes, it was a police cruiser. Tucker pulled over to the side and the police officer pulled over behind us and approached our car. She then knocked on the window and Tucker was like, "What's the problem, officer?" She replied, "You were speeding and swerving; where are you going in such a hurry?" I chimed in, saying that I had to poop and had told him to speed up. She smiled and let us go, saying to drive slowly and be safe.

Back at the house, we passed around the coffee and toasted bagels, not mentioning to my wife or Lizbeth what had just happened. My symptoms had momentarily disappeared from this excitement, but by the time our friends left for home a few hours later, my unsteadiness was back. Thinking about what this could mean gave me goosebumps; however, I tried not to show it.

I went to sleep that night with darkness in the window and woke up six hours later looking at my clock and realizing it was time for work. But the sunlight through the window looked brighter than usual. Again, I felt like I had been heavily drinking all night. I told my wife, and together we decided I would call in to work and tell them I would be out for the day. I then called our family doctor to explain my issue, and he set up an appointment for that afternoon.

CHAPTER 2

Doctors Know it All, Right?

We arrived at the doctor's office, and I was given some simple movement tests. I was asked to stand on one leg, which did not happen; I kept losing my balance. I was asked to walk backward, and I somehow managed to accomplish this task, although it took me longer than usual. My doctor sent me straight to a neurologist to dig deeper into what was going on. My hairs stood up and chills came over my body as I entered the neurologist's office. He began by hitting my knee with a rubber hammer to test my reflexes, touching my nose with my eyes closed, and testing my sensation by poking me in different places and having me guess where. I knew something was off when he sent me to the hospital for an MRI of my brain. My heart began to pound rapidly in my chest. The hospital was a few blocks away, and as I approached, I could feel the chills coming again, my heart beating faster and faster the closer I got to the hospital.

I entered the hospital and saw a washroom just inside the doors. Seeing a place that I could be alone, I stepped inside, went to the sink, and turned on the cold water. After splashing my face a few times, I gazed into the mirror and noticed that my face was pale. I turned off the water and dried my face with a paper towel. I looked in the mirror once more, closed my eyes, took a deep breath, and left the washroom. The elevator was right beside the washroom, so I pressed the up button.

I tapped my foot patiently as I waited, but I could feel the goosebumps forming. The elevator door opened, and I pressed the button for the second floor.

The elevator door closed, and the ride up felt like slow motion. It seemed to take 10 minutes to reach the second floor, but it must have been 10 seconds at most. The door opened, and I got out and strolled to the MRI department just a few meters ahead. I approached the secretary and informed her I was there for my brain scan. I was told to take a seat and I'd be called shortly. I sat down, my skin turning red, and grabbed a magazine to read, but before I could open it, I heard my name called. I followed the lady to a gray machine that took up about half the room. In the middle of it was a big tunnel with a place to lay down, and the lady told me to get inside. As soon as my head was resting on the pillow, I was pushed all the way inside the tunnel. The machine began to wind up and I could hear a small object circling my head. It was going faster and getting louder each time it went around, and sometimes it would make a knocking sound. My time in the MRI machine lasted for about 20 minutes. When the scan had finished, the sound gradually slowed until the machine was silent. The technician told me to get up and report back to the neurologist for the results. I did as I was told, my hands wet with sweat.

Once I was in front of the neurologist, my heart once again began to pound and crush against my ribs, but it felt like it was beating in slow motion. The neurologist looked at my MRI, pointing to a chart of the human brain hanging on the brown wall to show me that I had a cyst on my brain stem, just below the brain. He said that they do not operate on that site due to the risk involved. I felt frozen at that moment. I was confused and full of questions, but our meeting was over before I had a chance to ask any. It was only after I left, however, that the reality of the inoperable cyst began to sink in.

The only thing the doctor told me that I understood was that a nurse would visit me daily to check for any changes in my condition. I had no idea how to respond; all I could do was get into my car and start to drive. People were honking at me, but I did not hear. All I could think of was what was going to happen. How would I tell my wife and my parents? *This cannot be real*, I thought all through the long drive home.

Back home, I repeated what the neurologist had said to my wife. Even then, I did not fully grasp the seriousness of the situation and went about my life, telling myself that this situation wasn't dangerous. I let this positive thought drive out all the doubt in my mind, and as I repeated this mantra to myself over and over, I started to believe it.

The CD

A couple days later, I decided to get the brain images from the hospital to see for myself what this was about. Back at the same imaging office, the lady checked my identification and told me it would be $25 to get the CD with my brain scan images. I was told to come back the next day to pick it up. The next day arrived, the receptionist checked my identification once more, and I finally received my brain scan CD.

I found it very pleasing how easy it was to get access to my medical records. After receiving my CD, I drove back through the traffic and eventually got home. The minute my car was parked in the driveway, I ran downstairs to my computer and inserted the CD. I could not wait to see what the neurologist was talking about. After installing the necessary software to view the CD, I was finally able to see my brain for the very first time. Before me sat dozens of 3D images. I had no idea what I was looking at, but after patiently clicking through 30 of them, I saw something that looked like the shape of a brain.

Although I could now see my brain, I still had no idea what the neurologist was referring to since I could not distinguish the cyst from the various other objects in the brain. I was puzzled as the pictures did not resemble what I imagined a brain would look like. It took another 30 minutes before I finally recognized a huge bubble on the brain stem. If I could describe the location of the cyst, it would be in the back-middle-top of my neck, just below the base of the skull.

I honestly did not see any trouble with the location of this cyst and saw no reason why removing it would cause the kind of operational risk to my life that I had been warned of.

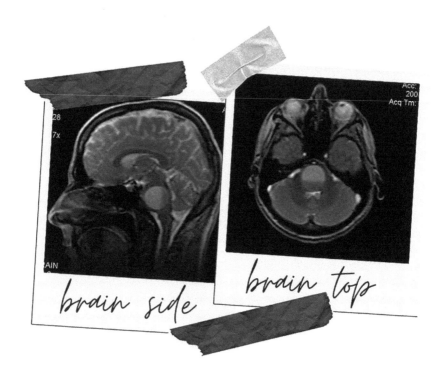

brain side   brain top

The next day, I noticed that my vision was weaker. This had been gradually getting worse for a few days and was really starting to bug me, so I made an appointment to get my eyes checked. This was late May 2008, and my parents had just gotten back from vacation. I normally worked with my dad and had been running the family business while he was away; a lot was new to me, but I had managed. When I saw my dad back at work, he commented that my speech was slurred, but I did not think much of it and went home like normal. The next day, I had double vision. Sometimes when I was reading my email, all the words appeared in a weaker ghost image on the left side.

The Failed Eye Cure Attempt

I went to a laser eye clinic for a free eye exam, thinking maybe lasers could fix my eye problem. I went to the lobby, and after a brief conversation with the secretary, waited for my name to be called. A lady came out and called my name, and we entered the room. I was told to sit in a chair with a gray machine at eye level attached to a handle that led to the ceiling, and she began testing my eyes. She put some weird drops in my eyes, and after the test told me to be seated back in the lobby and wait for 20 minutes. I picked up a magazine to read, but quickly put it down as my eyes could not focus on anything. Soon enough, my name was called again.

Back in the room, more tests were done on my eyes and then I was told to rest in the lobby once more. Thirsty, I crossed the lobby to a water cooler and got a cup, but when I placed it underneath the tap, I couldn't read the label so I just threw the cup in the garbage and flopped back down in my chair. 10 minutes later, I was called back in.

I was at the eye clinic for eight hours in all. I got called by a different lady, with curly blonde hair and perfume so strong you could taste it. I followed her into her office, my eyes squinting, and she explained the procedure they recommended, the risk involved, and the cost. My eyes went big when I heard the price and the risk, and I left the room with my teeth clenched tight.

Driving home, I could not read the road signs, just the colors. I think I got honked at, but I made it home. A few days later, my double vision was back; even when I was driving, I saw two lanes and two of every vehicle, but I told myself, *Whatever,* and went on with my business.

Getting Contacts

Next, I got my eyes checked by Dr. Devram. He did not find anything wrong with my eyes except weak eyesight and offered me the choice between glasses and contacts. I was afraid of glasses, don't know why, so I chose contacts. A few days passed, and it was time to pick up my contacts. Dr. Devram showed me how to insert them into my eyes and how to remove them. He then had me sit in a chair with a mirror in front of me, the contacts on the table, and practice removing and inserting them until I could do it comfortably. Once this became easy, I was able to leave.

With the contacts in, everything was back to normal, or so I thought. I left the optometrist's office with a satisfied grin on my face from having solved this problem.

The next day, however, I ate a banana and immediately felt like vomiting. During my lunch break at work, resting in my office after reviewing and pricing out different projects, the nausea got so bad that I needed to leave. My wife was working, and I did not want to be alone in my situation, so I went to my parents' house. I told my mom of my continuing unwellness and went to lie down after drinking a cup of tea, but I did not tell her the details of my situation. I did not want to worry her; plus, I was afraid of the information spreading and I did not feel up to explaining everything to more people. A few hours passed, and the nausea went away, so I went back home. Everything seemed normal for about two weeks, so when the nurse came each day -usually the same nurse—and asked if anything was different, I would say no. She was quite nice, but to me this seemed like a waste of time.

One evening, we had my parents over to our house for a late supper of baked pork with sauce. After dinner, we showed them my MRI images. But this caused unwellness in me, so I went to lie down. It was strange; I suddenly found myself unable to cope with multiple sounds, even numerous voices in a room, and would just need to get away from the noise. When I tried to ignore my body's feedback, the unwellness would just keep getting worse, and I would start to get dizzy. But after around 20 minutes of lying down, my symptoms disappeared. I drank some coffee, then rejoined my wife and parents on the living room couch where we discussed my situation for hours. Finally, seeing night outside the window, my parents realized it was time to go. After making me promise to keep them updated about my health, they left for home.

The next day, I told my doctor that I felt nauseous, and he told me to report to the same neurologist again. I drove slowly to his office, my skin turning red from nervousness and my hands getting sweaty in anticipation of the visit. When I told him what had been happening to me, I was sent for another picture of my brain. When I reported back, the neurologist told me the cyst had increased in size and they had no choice but to operate. With that news, I turned red instantly, and I could feel the sweat dripping underneath my T-shirt, my legs wanting to buckle, and my body shaking all over. I left the neurologist's office with watery eyes from barely suppressed crying. I did not know how to tell this news to my wife. I got into my car slowly, closed the door, and gradually put the key in the ignition. The car started to move, and I drove off ever so reluctantly, my head filled with thoughts of the operation.

When I got home, I was comforted to see the house nicely illuminated on the street. I parked in the driveway, getting out slowly; everything seemed to be happening in slow motion. I carefully turned the key in the front door to slow the time until I would need to report what I had been told at my appointment. Wobbly, and with watery eyes, I trudged up the stairs, dropped down on the couch, and with my voice cracking, called for my wife to tell her the news.

CHAPTER 3

Hospital Stay

We traveled the next day to Hamilton General Hospital and met with the surgeon who would be performing the operation. He looked at my brain scan images, then back at me. I had no desire for a repeat of what I had heard from the neurologist, especially with my wife sitting next to me, but he gave us the information anyway. I was then admitted to the hospital to spend the night before my surgery.

Late afternoon was all right at the hospital; I had the room to myself, and the nurse came every few hours to check things like my pulse and temperature. For one of the checks, I had to lift my right leg up. However, the nighttime was totally different. Imagine you are in bed, and each time you fall asleep, a nurse comes and wakes you up to check on you. This meant checking my pulse, my blood pressure, and everything else, even raising my right leg, and I am not exaggerating when I say this happened five times. I got no sleep that night.

In the morning, I had to mentally prepare myself for a tough conversation with my parents. I knew I had to tell them that if things went sour, they should go on without me. I realized this was a conversation I never really practiced, and every time these thoughts came into my head, my eyes would tear up and my forehead would begin to sweat. Still, I knew it had to be done.

My mom brought me beet juice to drink, and let me tell you, this was the worst aftertaste I ever had in my life. I could only manage a quarter of the glass before I had to put it down. I started my talk, and even though I had tried to prepare for it, I still felt color coming to my cheeks. My heart started beating faster, the tears appeared in my eyes, and in a quiet, cracking voice I was beginning to say the words I had been practicing, but I never had the chance to finish them because I was interrupted by my parents, who gave words of encouragement that could have come out of a movie: "Everything will be okay," and "There's nothing to worry about." This was a very emotional conversation, and although I tried, it was hard to keep the sadness off my face.

I do not remember everything that was said in that moment, but I do remember the hug and the bittersweet feeling at the end. After the conversation with my parents, my wife came in and gave me some more encouragement.

Then the surgeon came in and told me they could not go ahead with the operation because it was too dangerous, but they would continue to monitor me. With that, I was sent home. I was told this while sitting in bed in my blue hospital gown, and I must say this news gave me a strange mix of disappointment and relief.

Before heading home, I had another brain scan to see if any changes had occurred, and it showed the cyst had grown bigger once again. The neurologist was surprised that it had not burst yet; but still did not suggest doing anything about it. I could feel myself getting angry at their inaction as I left the doctor's office. I drove myself home, shaking and with my hands warm to the touch.

Time for a Second Opinion

My mother-in-law referred me to a neurosurgeon at St. Michael's Hospital in Toronto who might be able to give a second opinion since nothing was being done. I showed him the pictures from my MRI and asked what he would suggest. He told me to have a seat and he would present my two options. He would be able to remove the cyst, but the way it was done would be up to me. My eyes opened wide and I gave him my full attention to hear the choices.

There was an easier way which would cause more damage to me; I would not be able to walk, I would lose all sensation on my left side, the right side of my face would be paralyzed, and my coordination would be off. The second choice was harder to access but would result in less damage to me; maybe just some changes on the left side with some weakness in my left arm. If he was unsuccessful in eliminating the problem, he would just drain the cyst to relieve the pressure it was causing in my brain, and by the time it grew back, I would be in my nineties. With that information, the meeting ended, and I was left to think about my options.

CHAPTER 4

Fed Up

With these choices in mind, I started to take matters into my own hands by doing some research. When we got home from the doctor's, the first thing I did was sit down at the kitchen table, open my laptop, and begin to gather some information about the brain. I stumbled on an article that said if you do not consume fat, tumors and cysts cannot survive. This article got my attention and I read it a few times and did some further research. I noticed there was lots of positive feedback from people who had followed the article's recommendation.

Intrigued, I decided to eliminate some fat from my diet.

I went further and began reading books and magazines on the topic. I had enough of not knowing. Everything the doctors were telling me was gibberish, a language I did not understand. I turned red and got thirsty, so I got myself a glass of vodka, drank half, and then came straight back to my laptop to research some more.

I went back to the article about fat and read it a couple more times. There was a chart that told the amount of fat in many common food items, and you were not allowed to go over a certain amount per day. But I decided to go to the extreme and eliminate fat altogether. I started to eat only things that were green. In the morning I usually ate asparagus, and at lunch some green salad. Whenever I started to feel hungry,

I just ate celery to stop the hunger. I drank only water and consumed only green foods.

Meanwhile, I became deeply knowledgeable about the brain. I was finally able to read MRI scans and distinguish the parts of the brain and their functions. Even with no formal education in this area, I taught myself things that many doctors in the field are unaware of. I learned that there were other ways this surgery could take place, but that they would involve making an incision in parts of the brain that were not well documented. Surgeons only operate on parts of the brain that are fully understood to avoid damaging the brain. No one was willing to enter the unknown part even though it would have made the operation easier and safer. Knowing this made me angry. How can you make progress if you do not try?

The phone rang, it was my parents inviting us for steak dinner. Of course, we accepted, but I told them I could not eat meat and would explain later. The sun was bright and high in the sky, and you could feel the dryness in the air. We got into the car and my wife started passing other cars like we were late for an appointment. My parents met us in the driveway, and I briefly explained my situation, but not in detail— not wanting to worry them, I made up most of the story, but did explain the no-fat method. It was hard seeing everyone eating steak while I ate asparagus. Seeing and hearing the juicy steak being cut and chewed made me rethink everything. After I had washed down my green dinner with a glass of water, my wife and I headed home.

Let us just say after the second day on my new diet, my energy level dropped big time. But I did not let this discourage me. I kept on eating my asparagus, adding some butter and salt for flavor. I kept this up for about a week, but then I pooped green, which really freaked me out and that was it for this diet.

At this point, I decided it was time to take some time off work. I tried to tell the secretary what was happening, but I could not hold it together and burst into tears in front of her. She told me it would not be an issue because she would handle my phone calls. Taking the time off work helped me think about my situation and the things that I had to do. Let us just say that thinking about this sucked; I would rather have worked and been busy than think about my condition. I tried to occupy myself by doing things I liked, however, thoughts of my health never quite left me. They were always in the back of my mind, silently reminding me everything was not okay. Crazy thoughts about the worst-case scenario went through my mind. Just in case I did not make it, I prepared documentation for my parents: Internet passwords, online banking, home phone, internet provider, and so on. I wanted to make sure all the details of my life would be explained so they would not have a difficult time. With tears in my eyes, I also prepared a list of things that needed attention that I had not gotten to yet so I would not be leaving a mess if things went sour.

My monitoring schedule said I was to do another brain scan to see if anything had changed. This seemed repetitive and a complete waste of time; I already knew what the result would be. Comparing the images I'd already had, I knew the cyst would have grown once again.

In the meantime, anything that I consumed was vomited up and just made me red. On the way to the hospital for the brain scan, my wife drove fast and passed cars so we would get there before I got nauseous in the car, but we still had to stop so I could throw up. We pulled into a parking lot next to a blue car, and I am sure they had a nice surprise seeing my textured brown puddle of food chunks by the driver's door. We got back on the road, but once again the nausea came, and we stopped in a different parking lot. I swung the door open and you could see the redness on my face as I leaned out the door, but nothing happened. I waited a couple minutes to make sure, leaning out the door, but still nothing. I leaned back in my seat, closed the door, and told my wife to step on it before this occurred again.

As we approached St. Joseph's Hospital in Hamilton, I was wondering how I would be able to lie in the machine for 20 minutes for the brain scan to finish. In the lobby, I suddenly had the nauseous feeling again. I quickly jogged past all the people in the hallway, and not looking back, pushed my way into the washroom, closed the stall door, knelt by the toilet bowl, and put my head inside. But nothing happened. I waited for 10 minutes, then got up and went to my appointment on the second floor. Luckily, there was no one else in the elevator. I went straight to the window at the brain scan department and told the lady who I was. The machine was already set up and she escorted me to the machine. She could see my wobble, the redness and the sweat that had just started to appear. She helped me lie down in the machine, and as she pushed me inside the tunnel, I began to pray that I would not need to use the red "In Case of Emergency" button.

Luckily, I lasted the whole scan and even the drive home was uneventful.

A few days went by, and still I could not hold anything down. No matter what I tried to eat or drink, it all came back up in the toilet after five minutes.

You could now see redness constantly on my face, and my voice sounded firm. To get some nutrients into my body, I bought some energy liquids, energy bars, and multivitamins. *Something must stay down*, I thought. I started to question a lot of what the doctors had said, but my biggest question was why nothing was being done and they were just monitoring my situation until my body gave up.

Looking in the mirror that week, I started to see my bones. I was able to notice the dramatic changes that come with losing weight so rapidly—one day I was relaxing on the couch when the phone rang, and I tried to get up, but to my surprise, I couldn't even lift my body. I was confused, but on the second try I managed to get up and answer the phone. I walked to the bedroom to take a nap, and when I woke up, I saw stars out the window.

I slept until the sunrise was coming in the window, then started to get dressed. I swung my legs off the bed, planting my feet on the floor and trying to push myself up, but I could not do it. My heart started to pound rapidly in my chest, spots of blackness danced into my vision, and I started to twitch. After relaxing for five minutes in bed with a variety of thoughts going through my head, most of them negative, I gave it another try.

I started to put on socks first, which meant reaching down to the floor, but looking this way made me see objects moving everywhere. I raised my head up to resume my sitting position on the side of the bed, stopped everything, and just looked at the wall, praying for my vision to return to normal. I stayed quiet, not wanting to wake my wife, who was in bed beside me. After I had stared at the wall for 10 minutes, everything returned to normal and I got up.

I remember we had some people over later in the afternoon, and I started being very wobbly and once again slurring my words as if I had been drinking heavily. I could not pay attention to anything that was happening, and the multiple voices and other noises jumbled together in my head. Trying to focus on one just gave me a headache. After 10 minutes of this, I decided to lie down. I walked to my bedroom, red in the face, and slammed the door behind me. On the bed, I squeezed the pillow between my hands in frustration and kicked the blanket upward, my heels coming down on the mattress several times. Then I closed my eyes and fell asleep, but I woke to light shining on my face through the window. At least my symptoms were gone when I got up. I felt kind of rude for taking a nap when I had guests over, but they understood my situation and no feelings were hurt.

CHAPTER 5

Healer Is a Joke

Soon after this, I heard that a healer was in town—someone who could heal with his hands. I had always been very skeptical of anyone who claims this ability, but I decided to give it a try since nothing else was happening. My wife took me to my first appointment with him; I quickly explained my situation, then he had me sit down on a chair and placed his hands on my head. To be honest, I never felt any warm sensation like people often claim to experience when being healed, and I felt no different after our session. Still, I was optimistic and agreed to come back the next day. I visited this healer three times in our city, then he went back to Toronto and told me to visit him there.

My close friend, Leszek Lasinski, drove me to Toronto and we chatted about the healer on the way. Like me, he was skeptical, but we were both curious to see what would happen. When we finally got to his office, I flopped down on a chair, and the treatment continued. But the healer only placed his hands on my head for about a minute before my session was over. I started to question whether we had come all this way for nothing, but I kept silent because some part of me still believed this could help and I wanted to continue. On my third visit, I was very wobbly and slurring my words heavily—and I mean heavily—as soon as I got out of the car. I started up the stairs to the healer's office, holding tightly to the handrail, thinking I might drop at any moment, but

I managed to hang on and made it for the treatment. After my friends took me home this time though, I decided to stop this nonsense. I was getting worse and not better. Alone in my bedroom, the full weight of this situation that no one else seemed to comprehend came crashing down on me, and I sobbed as I sat on my bed.

My wife's friend told me about another healer, claiming he had cured her of cancer. I was very skeptical of this, but in my situation, I thought, *What the heck, I will try it.* This was close to Toronto, and to get to this man's office I had to walk up two flights of stairs, holding the handrail tightly and not looking down. By the time I made it to the lobby, sweat had broken out on my forehead and I had to take three rest breaks. I told the receptionist I had arrived, then noticed that the other people waiting all had some form of pills in their hands. I wondered what these could be for. After a brief wait in the lobby, I was called in to see the healer. I explained my situation, and he told me to sit down in the chair. As soon as he placed his hands on my head, this experience began to resemble my previous one. *This is full of baloney*, I found myself thinking, but I kept quiet. He kept his hands on my head for about three minutes, after which he grabbed a vibrating machine and vibrated my neck and head. The whole time, I was wondering how this could possibly help me. He vibrated for about two minutes, then gave me some vitamins to take and some herbal tea to drink. Of course, I felt no different. As I left the office, looking back at all the people who had been suckered into buying pills, I knew I would not be coming back. To me, it seemed he was scamming these poor people who needed help and fell for this kind of stuff by claiming that he could heal.

The next morning, which was a Saturday, I was lying on the couch and saw out the window that my wife was washing the car in the driveway. Thirsty, I got up for a glass of water, then flopped back down and turned the TV on. Five minutes later, like an old familiar routine, the nausea came. I stood from the comfortable couch, walked over to the washroom, opened the door, put my head in my toilet bowl, and got into the vomiting position. From my throat came the sounds of vomiting and I was sure something would come out, but nothing happened. With my head in the toilet bowl, I shook my head and told myself I could not live like this. At that moment, I decided to do the freaking surgery. I no longer cared what happened. At this point, I had just had enough of what was happening to me.

Decision Made

I went out to the driveway and told my wife that the nausea had come back, and I had decided to do the surgery at St. Michael's Hospital. We got into the car and headed for Toronto. On the way there, my worries seemed to disappear and for a moment I forgot where we were going. I was feeling free, blasting the car radio, and singing along.

But there were other thoughts going through my mind as we got closer to the hospital. As I looked out at all the cars and people, I was thinking it was nice to finally not have to worry, to have come to a decision. I told myself this was what had to be done. But let us be honest, it was hard to not be nervous about the impending surgery.

All through the drive to Toronto, I felt normal, like there was nothing wrong with me, but I did not let this feeling fool me one bit. We arrived at St. Michael's Hospital and booked in with the doctor. They ran some tests, then told me I had the choice of spending the night in the hospital or going home and monitoring my situation there. With everything that had already happened though, the decision was easy: I just wanted to get this over with. I told them that I would spend the night there, and then first thing in the morning, be cured of this cyst in my head that had turned my life into a nightmare.

I remember lying in a single bed in a room with square white tiles on the ceiling and curtains that I could pull all around my bed. I remember the clock hanging on the white wall and noticing that it only took a few hours for the day to turn into evening. I hugged my wife, telling her to go get some sleep and that I would see her tomorrow. My daughter was with my in-laws that weekend, so I knew she was taken care of and I tried to sleep.

I slept for maybe an hour until the police brought in some drunk fellow who would not stop swearing. Every sentence he uttered had one or more swear words, and he was not cooperating one bit. Finally, they managed to get him into bed, telling him he needed to go to sleep, but he got out of bed every few minutes, bothering the nurses and swearing at them. My room was nearby and the door to the hallway was wide open, so I heard everything. Finally, after two hours of this, the police handcuffed him to the bed, but he still would not stop swearing. Forget about sleep. I think finally they put him to sleep by injecting him with a sedative, but this was early in the morning.

Later in that long early morning, I heard some ladies and then another man being escorted in by the police. Once again, I could hear everything they said. It was an interesting night—I certainly did not get much sleep—and I am sure things were even more interesting for the hospital staff.

CHAPTER 6

First Surgery

When the morning sun hit my face, my condition felt even worse, but it was finally time for the surgery. A nurse rolled me in my bed to the operating room, where I could see the surgeon looking over my blue-tinted MRI images hanging on the wall and discussing the procedure with his staff.

Meanwhile, the two nurses who were setting things up for the surgery asked me if I needed assistance getting onto the flat metal operating table. Beside the table was an impressive amount of machinery, an IV, and some surgical tools. All of this took place within maybe one minute, and I was not able to memorize all the details. I got onto the table, they hooked up the IV to my arm, then connected me to the machine with some white stickers on my body. I remember taking one last look at the door, and then I was asleep.

When I opened my eyes, I was in complete darkness. I heard the nurse's voice telling me not to touch my head, but I couldn't resist; I needed to touch my head, like a child who is told not to press the red button suddenly wants nothing more than to press the red button. So, I had to constantly fight the temptation not to touch my head.

The nurse told me that the surgery had been successful, and I know she could see my eyes start to water. Just then, my parents and my wife entered the room.

I do not remember everything that was said, I just remember a warm hug from my mom and a kiss on the cheek. A few minutes later, they were told to leave so that I could rest. The nurse had probably noticed my droopy eyes that I had fought to keep open and the sweat that had dampened the bed. Once they left, I noticed that my left arm had a strange tingly feeling, kind of like an army of ants walking down it. I raised my arm to see if everything was okay, but when I tried to put it down, I hit my face. I repeated this process a few times, not hitting my face anymore, but then the nurse came and told me to go to sleep. It was then that I noticed the darkness outside; the surgery must have lasted all day. I put my arm down and closed my eyes. *This is not so bad; I can deal with some weakness and tingling in my left arm.*

I should say that much of this information comes from my parents; I have almost no recollection of those first few hours after surgery. It was a weird feeling, and I have an idea now of what it must be like to lose your memory. Apparently, the surgeon was not able to eliminate the source of the cyst; instead, he drained it like we had discussed earlier.

Confused About Second Surgery

I awoke in a different post-op room; now there were two nurses walking around checking on me, and my parents do not recall any other patients being in the room. I was lying in bed, talking with my parents about the surgery in a normal voice. This room had a window, through which I could see the roofs of other buildings and the bright light of the sun. But before I could admire the view, I suddenly started choking. My parents called for a nurse, who called three other medical personnel into the room. Together they began to hit me on the back so I could breathe. But my bodily functions were shutting down one by one. I was then rushed for an emergency surgery, and since my original surgeon was out of the country, it was done by a different surgeon. This surgeon decided to take the route with easier access to the source of the problem but more potential for damage that would occur. As I was falling into a coma and my whole body was shutting down, it was a quick life-or-death decision with no time to hesitate or think about the consequences.

After this second surgery, I opened my eyes for a moment and saw shapes that must have been my wife, my in-laws, and my parents standing around my bed. I could somewhat distinguish the shapes, but I could not see the details to know who each shape belonged to. My skin was red, and my forehead was sweating; when I tried to speak, no words came out, only sounds. Even when I tried to move my arms, I found them pinned to the bed by their own weight.

I was placed in the ICU to monitor my progress. This room was dark and sunless, and my parents do not recall any other patients there. The first evening after the surgery, the nurses saw that there was sweat covering my body and turned on a fan on my right side, pointing it toward my head. Unfortunately, I was unable to fully close my right eye and it began to dry out. Thankfully, my parents lowered my eyelids down, but in the morning the nurse forced my right eyelid up, ripping some of the cornea.

When I awoke, I could see that my parents had been crying. My father-in-law went to grab my daughter Isabella so I could see her, and I would never forget the moment she touched my forehead and said, "Daddy's all wet." I could not stop looking at her. A machine started to beep because my blood pressure had instantly gone up, and the nurse said to take Isabella away. My eyes stayed on her as she was taken out of the room, she was slowly getting smaller and smaller until she was gone. Once she was out of the room, my blood pressure went back to normal. But after a few minutes, everyone was told to leave so I could rest.

I was under a lot of medication, so the details are a bit of a blur here. Because the incision to the cyst was from the right side of the brain, this surgery left me quite disabled. I could no longer walk or write, had extreme muscle weakness with the left side being more severe, saw double, couldn't feel my left side, my coordination was extremely off, and my speech was reduced to a mumble. I could no longer eat, and the right side of my face was paralyzed; I could not even blink my right eye. All because a rash decision was made to go with this surgery, which left me with all the symptoms my wife and I had been warned about at St. Michael's Hospital.

CHAPTER 7

Recovery

Although I was under lots of medication, I do vaguely remember my friend, Vlad Spehar, visiting me on Sunday in my room. I believe he gave me a funny book with cartoony pictures of people sitting on the toilet. I was in a 10' x 20' room with a window on the side of the wall which I could neither reach nor see through. My bed had white sheets and a blue blanket, the lights were dimmed about halfway, and there was a door a couple of feet beyond the bed. The nurses were changing constantly, making it impossible to remember any of their names. There was a bit of redness on my face, and Vlad could see some droplets of sweat on my forehead like I had been working out. My eyes were droopy and not fully opened; I would try to talk to visitors like Vlad by mumbling, and although it sounded correct in my head, I'm sure they didn't understand a word of my gibberish.

My wife and parents arranged to take turns visiting me. My parents would come in the afternoon and my wife in the morning, and Isabella would stay with my in-laws. I would like to thank my mom here for visiting me each of those days from early in the morning to late in the afternoon; I know this was difficult since my parents lived 45 minutes out of Toronto and she usually had to take the train to see me. It was genuinely nice to have some company instead of being alone. In moments like these, scared and defenseless, you do not want to be alone.

The surgery left me so weak that I could not even make a sound. My parents brought a big letter board with big colorful letters and numbers that I could point at to communicate—at least, that was the idea. I had no clue how little strength I had in my arms until I attempted to point at a letter. My first time attempting this task, I extended my left index finger and, clenching my fist with the effort, began to lift my left arm. I focused intently on the letter, but as soon as my hand reached it, my arm fell back onto the bed.

My forehead was covered with sweat, my face was red, and I was breathing heavily, but I was determined. I practiced pointing vigorously at anything in the room, even the Kleenex box. My goal was to be able to point at a letter on the next attempt, and when my mom visited, she would help me point to various items around the room. I was adamant that I would succeed in this task.

Pointing took a while to get good at. Finally, I got to where I could finish half a word; my favorite letters on the board were I, L, and U. These got pointed to a lot; however, I was never able to really finish a word before my arm got too tired out. But I learned to point to enough letters that the people around me could finish the sentence for me. After a few days of communicating this way, my speech slowly started to come back. It was mostly mumbling, but I was able to say first letters, then words, around 10% of which were understood. This made communicating a lot easier.

In the evening, around 7 p.m. by the clock above me on the wall, the nurses moved me to a wheelchair. Although the bed was reasonably comfortable with two pillows a semi-soft mattress, I could not be in bed the whole time. Usually two nurses assisted me into the wheelchair and wheeled me in front of the TV, handing me the remote and a red button I could press if I needed assistance.

I found it very strange that I could not adjust myself in the wheelchair. I wanted to lift myself higher, so I called the nurse by pressing the button and told her that all I needed was help adjusting my position and a pillow to hold my head up—my head was heavier than I could ever have imagined. Soon, I began to get unbelievable body pain every time I was in the wheelchair for more than 15 minutes. My head never really hurt, but the body pain was intense, and I pressed the red button to call the nurse. Once she arrived, I explained that the extreme pain was in my lower back, hips, legs, and the top of my arms. She gave me morphine, and in one minute the pain disappeared.

Morphine is hard to describe, but I will try. Since I already had an IV, the drug was injected into the tube that was connected to the needle in my vein. When the morphine hit my blood vessel, a warm sensation blossomed at the point of insertion and instantly began to spread throughout my body. All my pain was suddenly gone, and I had a serene feeling of comfort for about ten minutes. It felt so good that as it started to wear off, I pressed the button to get more. Of course, I no longer had pain, but when the nurse arrived, I told her the pain was back. But this time she gave me Tylenol 3 instead. It felt like nothing compared to the morphine, and I felt sad. I understand, though, that they did not want to get me addicted to morphine.

Head Lift

My parents came into the room with the next morning's sun. They wanted to take me out to the hospital lobby, so they called the nurses, who transferred me into the wheelchair. Once the nurses left, my dad approached and stood at the back of the wheelchair and pushed me out the door and into the hallway.

On my right, I could see a couple of nurses walking by and doors leading to other rooms. I felt a warmth coming over my body, like being in the sun. I touched my forehead with my hand, and it felt funny. Bringing my hand down to my face, I saw it glistened with moisture. I rolled my eyes and wiped my hand on the hospital gown I was wearing but said nothing. At the elevator, I saw we were on the seventh floor. My parents pressed the down button.

The elevator arrived, and we had it to ourselves. The door closed, they pressed the button for the first floor, and we started to go down. The lights went out and when they came back on, we were in the lobby. My senses were bombarded with things I knew I could not have; my mom ordered juice, and I watched longingly as she drank it through a white straw, but I resisted the temptation to ask for some.

I wanted to lift my head, but it surprised me by immediately dropping back down and hitting the head support on the wheelchair. I was confused about what had just happened; I tried again, this time timing myself on the clock on the wall above the order desk. This time I managed to keep my head up for ten seconds. I could not believe that my head was so heavy; I had never thought about this, but who does? I mentioned this to my parents, showing them how I would lift my head and it would drop after just five seconds, and they were as surprised as I was. But I was determined to change this. My parents took me back to the room and left me in the wheelchair, but I started to practice lifting my head.

When the sunlight hit my face the next day, my parents showed up again and took me to the lobby like before. I wanted to show them that I could hold my head up for five minutes before it dropped on the headrest. In the lobby, my mom ordered another juice and they sat down at a table next to the wall. I raised my voice to get their attention. "Look at me!" I said as I began to lift my head. I could feel the redness on my face, but my head was lifted. I turned left and right, my head still up and not dropping like the day before. In my mind I could see the grin that was forming on my face, and my parents were surprised at this quick development. I am sure they did not understand my mumble, but I told them, "You will see me walk again."

CHAPTER 8

The Outside World

The next morning, my wife asked for permission to take me outside since it was a nice sunny day. Permission was granted, and after three nurses transferred me from my bed into a wheelchair, my wife pushed me outside. Across the street from the hospital were a park, a little church, and a small mall. The mall seemed out of place, but the park looked perfect for someone who wanted to relax. We went to the park first and spent a few good hours there watching the birds flying between the treetops. I wanted to visit the church, which looked old and was decorated with statues on the side, but for some reason it was closed every time we tried to go there. The next day, my parents took me back to the park, and we spent quite a bit of time there. They took me to the middle of the park and sat down on a brown bench where you could sprinkle some crumbs on the ground, and birds would come down and feast. It was genuinely nice to see life going on outside, and, of course, it beat being inside the hospital. My attention kept being drawn to the passing cars; they were a welcome break from the motionless white walls of my hospital room.

The evenings at the hospital were quite boring. Around 7 p.m. every day, two or three nurses transferred me into my wheelchair and placed me in front of the TV, which was about three feet to the right of the bed. After turning on the TV, the nurses would leave, but it only took 15 minutes of watching the news before I would get multiple kinds of pain all over my body, just like I did every time I sat in one position without moving. I planted my hands beside my hips and tried to lift my body to get deeper into the wheelchair, but I could not lift myself. I would call the nurse back to transfer me into the bed. There I would be comfortable and free from pain, covered in softness and sinking into the mattress, which was a gift from heaven. I knew this was not the best for my recovery, but I could not bring myself to care as I was comfortable and had the remote control in my hand.

I turned off the TV, but my eyes were still wide open. I grabbed the pillow to my face so the darkness could make me close my eyes. But my eyes were still open, staring into the pillow. I struggled and screamed into the pillow, hitting the mattress with my hands with all my energy. My breathing became fast and I could feel redness coming over my face. After a few minutes of this agony, I became droopy, my breathing and heartbeat slowed, and I fell asleep. When I opened my eyes, I could see that the clock above me had moved. My heart was hitting my chest, and I could hear its pounding along with the sound of the wind outside, but I could not see anything but the clock. I could not defend myself in this state, so I called the nurse. She came and turned on the light and saw that my face was full of sweat, my eyes were wide open, and I was crushing the pillow beside me. She then asked if I was okay, and with some confusion I answered, "I am now." Little did she know how real this experience had been to me.

When the morning sunlight hit my face, my wife showed up, and noticing my sweaty body, asked if everything was okay. I could not answer; there was something holding my lips together and keeping me from repeating what I had experienced earlier. I kept quiet, afraid to bring up my dream.

My wife called the nurse to move me into the wheelchair, then proceeded to push me out of the room, through the hallway and past the other rooms to the elevator, then through the lobby, and finally outside. We decided to change things up and visit the mall; it was a good change of scenery from the birds and trees in the middle of the park.

I could see the wheels on my wheelchair rolling forward fast, and I felt bad for being pushed all the time, but I was afraid that anything I said might come out the wrong way so I kept quiet, just feeling the sunlight on my face. This adventure was new to me, but I did not like being dependent on someone for a basic need like getting around. We opened the door to the mall and suddenly right in front of me was a big mirror. I looked at myself for the first time in days and immediately broke into tears, not comprehending what I saw. No words came to my mouth. It was like I was looking at the reflection of another person. Staring at my crooked face with my eyes wide open and a Band-Aid on my head, I tried to smile, but I could only see the left side move and the expression resembled nothing like a smile. This was the hardest thing I had been asked to accept so far; even as I type this, I find it exceedingly difficult to talk about. Words cannot really describe what it felt like to see myself in the mirror that day. I could not bear to look at myself anymore, and with tears in my eyes, I told my wife to turn me around. As we kept going through the mall, I fought to accept that the reflection I had seen was my own.

After my experience with the mirror, we went down the handicap path and into a cell phone store. I looked around at a few different cell phones before grabbing one that I had told my wife I would get when I got out, then told her I wanted to return to my room.

Once I was in my room, the physical therapist arrived. She had shoulder-length brown hair, and she took me to a machine next to the wall that I was to stand on. It had two-foot pedals that you stood on, and you got strapped in like you were wearing a diaper and held onto a bar with each hand for balance. The lady could control how much weight each foot pedal took, so I did not have to put my full weight on my feet. It felt incredible to stand for the first time since my surgery, and I smiled because I wanted more. Unfortunately, 10 minutes was all she had. I was subdued as I came down from the machine, disappointed that this had ended before any sweat had formed on my brow or any color had come to my face. She told me I had been putting my full weight on the machine, but I had seen that it was only 60%. I was impatient to try it again so I could put more weight on my feet.

Saliva

One time when my wife visited, she pointed out that I had saliva dripping down the right side of my lips. I couldn't feel anything, but now that she mentioned it, I looked down and saw a trail of saliva coming out from my mouth, slowly going down and pooling at the tip of my chin until it started to drip and form a wet spot on my leg. Apparently in my condition I was nearly unable to swallow my saliva, so I was given a plastic suction tube like a straw with one end connected to a hose. You could always hear the suction in the straw, and I started to check my face on a regular basis to make sure nothing was dripping. If there was anything, I would suck it away. I never knew how much saliva the body can produce, and it had to be sucked out every few minutes.

At one point, I suddenly realized I was never hungry anymore, which was strange. I believe this was when a feeding tube was inserted so they could control my appetite with liquid food.

One day when the sunlight woke me up, I remembered that it was my wife's birthday. A couple hours later, the nurse told me that I would be transferred to Hamilton General Hospital in Hamilton, Ontario. This was extremely exciting news since that hospital was close to home and my parents' house. When my wife arrived, I told her I had a birthday gift for her. I was not sure if she would understand this, but I proceeded to tell her the news of my transfer and this was exciting for her indeed. My wife told my parents not to come that afternoon since I would be transferred in a few hours.

CHAPTER 9

Going to Hamilton General Hospital

I do not really recall how I ended up in the transfer ambulance; I just remember it was somewhat of a long ride to the hospital. With every bump the ambulance went over, I felt like I was falling out of bed, and I grabbed hold of the bed. My heart was crashing against my chest, and I wished we would get there sooner. Finally, I could feel the ambulance slowing down and turning left, then it stopped, and my breathing slowed down to normal.

I remember being rolled into my new room; I had it all to myself and there were three channels on the TV, which hung right above the bed from a big gray pipe. My parents and my wife were there to greet me. Unfortunately, I was not able to drink the coffee they had brought, but the letter board I mentioned earlier had traveled with me. I often used it to communicate when my attempts at speech were not understood. If no one had any idea what I was saying, the pointing began and let me tell you, this was quite a workout. So, most of the time when I had visitors, I only spoke when I absolutely had to, knowing that pointing would be involved and this would just exhaust my strength.

When I transferred to the new hospital, I decided that I would also start a new routine., Each morning around 11, I got put into my wheelchair and sat facing the window next to my bed, where I could see the road through my window. There was not much to look at, but at least it was a change of scenery. Each long weekend that came it rained, and I found myself thinking that if I had to stay inside, at least the inclement weather was keeping others from going outside, too. I find that thought funny now.

Throat Hole for Safety

The doctors wanted to drill a small hole in my throat at the base of my neck to prevent me from choking; they said it was a precautionary measure just in case my symptoms returned. My wife and I were very skeptical of an unnecessary hole being drilled in me just above my ribcage, but they kept telling us how important the procedure was, and finally I gave the go-ahead. There was a small plastic tube with a lid, and if I closed the lid, I would soon start to choke. When I first put my hand to the tube and felt a constant rush of air blowing out, it made me jerk back in surprise. I was instructed to try and close the tube until it would stay closed, so as I lay in bed, I began to practice closing the tube with my finger. At first, I would start coughing after just five seconds. It took me a few days, but eventually, after hours of diligent practice, I succeeded in breathing with the tube closed.

It is a good thing I did, because when the tube was open, I could not speak. If I wanted to talk to anyone, I would need to close the tube. Then I would be able to use my voice, pointing to my loving letter board for assistance.

The mornings, late afternoons, and evenings were quite interesting. When I was placed in bed, I always watched the Food Network. I watched it so much that I started to remember how to bake, steam, boil, and fry several different foods. The funny part is that I still use some of those recipes to this day and even shared a few with my parents. So, in a way, this was a very educational time for me. This went on for a few days, as it was really the best channel available.

Right Eye Check

I was woken from sleep by the sound of footsteps entering my room. Opening my eyes and turning my head to the right, I looked toward the door and saw a man walk in. He introduced himself as an eye doctor and said that he wanted to see what could be done about my right eye. As you will remember, the right side of my face was paralyzed by the damage I sustained in surgery, and I was left unable to blink my right eye. This period is a little fuzzy since it happened such a long time ago; however, I do have some recollection of what came next.

Occasionally, I would be taken to a lower floor of the hospital without leaving my bed. I would be rolled out of my room, down the hallway, and into an elevator that could fit an entire bed. This was one of those times. The optometrist pressed the lobby button, and I felt the elevator sinking. We then exited and proceeded down the hallway, which was quite busy with nurses.

In the room he took me to, there was a different eye doctor; he tried to pop a few contacts into my eye, however, my memory is cloudy on why he was doing this. When he placed the contact lens in my right eye, I tried to close it, but this was still not possible. There was always a space that I could see through. I seem to recall a few more eye doctors visiting me over the following days, but I do not really remember what was done to me.

Hallway in the Hospital?

After the eye doctor left, I was rolled away and put next to the nurse that had black eyes, black hair down to her shoulders, and a gentle smile. From the clock on the wall to my right, it seemed that I waited there for a few hours.

Then I was in bed staring at the ceiling and noticed it was moving. Turning my head as much as I could, I saw I was in a hallway, and then I felt a needle pierce my skin and inject me with something. I saw that we passed through a big steel door, and I was rolled further down the hallway. No one else was in the hallway, just me and the moving ceiling. I saw my parents—we were having dinner and I was making toast—then I opened my eyes and saw a nurse. She took the blanket off me, and you could see the sweat on my forehead and the redness on my face. Looking around the room with my half-opened eyes, I saw that no one was there and closed my eyes again.

CHAPTER 10

Pee I Think

I woke to the sunlight in my face, and when I touched the blanket, my hand came away wet. My eyes opened wide, and I called the nurse and told her of the wetness. She cleaned it up, but on the way out of my room she slinked through the doorway with her eyes wide open.

The next morning, the blanket was wet again, but I had no idea what had happened. Confused, I called the nurse. When she strutted into my room, I told her about the wetness, and she said that a diaper would be put on me if it happened again. I went silent and a red look came over me. At least I knew now that I had peed myself in the night. Not knowing had been a very strange and confusing feeling. Apparently one of the medications I was on made me pee myself whenever I went into a deep state sleep. To this day, the need to pee when I sleep has never left me. At least now I do not wet myself, just wake up with the urge to pee.

I tried investigating all the medications I was on, but none listed this as a possible side effect. I even tried reflexology, acupuncture, and some herb therapies, but none of them worked. Over the years I accepted this, and it does not bother me as much as it used to, my sleep just sucks since I wake up a few times every night with the urge to pee.

The next day, a few friends came to visit. My friend, Artur Lasinski, gave me a few DVDs to watch if I got bored. I spent a few days at the hospital in my room, and one afternoon the physical therapy lady showed up and told me we would be starting PT and that she would come and get me in the morning.

The Stroll to Start Recovery

I was extremely excited to start physical therapy since I had not actually stood on my feet since my first surgery. Let us just say I was like a kid who knows they are getting the thing they have been wanting all year for Christmas. In the morning, when the physical therapist showed up, I was so anxious to start PT that I was already in my wheelchair waiting for her. As she pushed me away down the hallway, I felt like a kid on their way to get something they really want. Down the hall we went, then turned left and there it was: a high table with wheels on the front and normal legs on the back. She placed me behind the table and asked me to stand up. Standing in that moment was the most exciting thing that had happened to me in days, like a child getting a lollipop. Here I was, standing tall for the very first time! I was a bit unsteady and had to use the table for balance, but it felt like getting a good grade on a test. I was enormously proud of myself and could feel dampness in my left eye.

I looked at my physical therapist for further instructions. This task had been amazingly easy to accomplish without help. Sure, I had stood before, but not on my full weight. The physical therapist told me to lean on the table and start to move forward, looking straight ahead at my destination, which was my room. I lifted my right foot off the floor, thinking, *This is simple; nothing has changed.* I stepped forward proudly, but my left foot was dragging, and the placement was totally off.

No big deal, I thought to myself. *My left foot's just dragging a little.* The physical therapist put a plastic bag on my left shoe, which made my left foot more slippery. I stood up again and was ready for action, but once again my foot went inward. I was confused; this was not the placement I had been trying for. *No big deal*, I thought again. *I must be rusty.* I then placed my left foot in the correct position so I could move my right foot, but the same thing happened with my right foot. I looked at the physical therapist with disappointment in my eyes—like the child had opened the Christmas present, but it was not what they were expecting.

She encouraged me to try again, but still my feet disobeyed me and went inward. This devastated me, and I plopped back down in the wheelchair and asked to be pushed back to my room. Once I was in my room and the physical therapist left, I started to cry, silently so as not to make a scene. I thought to myself that this would take longer than I had thought, the surgery had left me a total mess. I was very heartbroken and just let this sink in for a good few hours, looking out the window as I sat in my wheelchair and pondered the future. I was overwhelmed and could no longer feel the drive to push myself that had been there just a few hours before. I pondered for quite a while, and while I was thinking, a picture came into my head. Snow was coming down heavily, and I was building a snowman and making snow angels with my daughter. In that moment, I promised myself that this image would become reality. This image remains my motivation to this day, whenever I feel down and things feel hopeless.

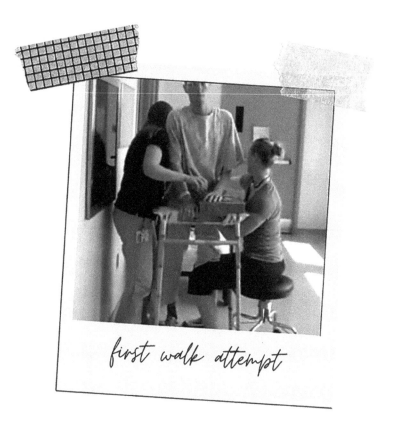

first walk attempt

I attempted to walk again the next day. It was not pretty, and I almost cried, but I did not. Instead I shut my teeth together hard and kept trying, mistake or not. I had cool glasses which somewhat covered my right eye to eliminate the double vision I was having, and it's still true to this day: the more obstruction to my right eye, the less double vision I have.

My PT lasted from the time it took me to walk from the PT room, through the hallway, and back to my room—around 30 minutes. At the end, I was red in the face, and you could see the droplets of sweat prickling my forehead. I did this a few days, of course.

I started asking anyone who had any kind of medical or PT experience how long they thought my recovery might take. The answers I got—some said I would be fully recovered in a few months—makes no sense now when I look back on it, but I will never forget what one man said. I met him one day while walking with the physical therapist; he asked what had happened to me, why I could not walk. My physical therapist answered that I had a brain operation. The man then explained that he had a stroke that had rendered him unable to eat, however, this was his last day, and he could not wait to eat a big steak. This reminded me that I had not eaten anything since the surgery, and it would be nice to have the taste of steak in my mouth.

I was doing very well with my physical therapy, and I got to a point where I was no longer fatigued after my walk to my room. So I began to think to myself that maybe this recovery would not take too long since I was already developing the strength needed for walking.

One day in the late afternoon, I was rolled in my bed to the MRI to see if my cyst was returning. But I did not know this at the time. I started to look around and ask where I was going, but no one would answer my questions. I started to mumble words to the men pushing my bed; however, I got no answer, and I was probably not understood anyway. I was gripping the bedsheet tightly, and I gnashed my teeth together so hard you could hear grinding.

I was taken to a scanning machine where they injected some liquid in my veins and then placed me in the machine, which was huge—I mean it took up like half the room. As I lay on my back in the machine, part of the machine started to move. A big arm was swinging in circles close to my head, and I thought it was going to hit my head. About two minutes later, I felt bad, and I mean bad, like something was going to turn out terribly. I still had no idea what was happening or why I was being scanned again. Then I opened my eyes and saw from the TV in front of my face and the picture of my daughter pinned to the wall, that I was back in my room. Out the window, I saw stars and streetlights, and the clock showed 11 p.m.

30 minutes later, I was rolled again in my bed to what I think was the main lobby, where all the nurses were gathering around and looking at me. I then closed my eyes.

When I opened my eyes, I could see the TV again in front of me. I threw off the blanket and started to grind my teeth, grabbing the mattress tight. I was visited by another nurse, but still no one would answer my questions, so I again closed my eyes.

My wife showed up and I opened my eyes when I heard a voice. I could see a different machine scanning my head as I lay in bed. After the scan was done, the nurse started placing white stickers onto my head. Finally, the doctor came and explained to my wife what was happening. From my understanding, the cyst had returned and was even bigger than before. I had been passing out, and they had been keeping me in the dark to avoid any complications that stress might bring. But the doctor told my wife that I was to be operated on immediately using the machine, which would be guided by the white stickers on my head.

3rd Surgery

Before any decision was made, I had a minor surgery to drill a small hole in my skull and relieve the pressure that the cyst was putting on my brain.

I opened my eyes and saw the letters ICU above me. My parents had arrived, but I was drifting in and out of consciousness. I remember being in the ICU a while. A person with a black gown and a cross necklace came to my bedside. He said a prayer, took my confession, and then left. My mom's friend worked at the hospital and she was in possession of a handkerchief that had belonged to our past pope John Paul II. I recall her wiping my face with the handkerchief, and then I was slowly rolled away in my bed. With watery eyes, my mom said, "We'll see each other in a few hours."

I did not know what was happening; nobody had told me anything, which made me very confused. I was rolled into a room with a small number of people dressed in blue. I believe I was placed on my back on a steel table, and I saw something like a bright figure in the back of the room that I could not quite make out, then I passed out.

I opened my eyes and could see my parents and my wife beside my bed. Finally, they explained to me everything that had happened. Originally, I was going to be operated on in the morning. Due to the challenging location and the fact that I had already had two surgeries awfully close together, my survival rate would be around 2%; however, if I were not operated on, it would be 0%. The surgeon didn't want to operate, but after a few hours had passed and he'd had time to think, he informed my wife and my parents that he would try to operate and remove the source of this cyst. He told them very simply that if nothing were done immediately, I would not survive the night and that the surgery was worth the risk. "I'll do it," he told them.

Of course, the lack of information to me was to keep me relaxed and not panicking in my sensitive state. Even with those slim odds, I survived the surgery. After this surgery, my recollection was a bit blurry; keep in mind that I was on a lot of medications, which I do not even recall being given to me.

CHAPTER 11

New Room, Strange Dreams

Although I do not remember it happening, I was rolled into a different room, larger than my previous one. This room had two levels, the top level about a meter higher than the bottom level, and on the left side was a handicapped walkway that they could use to roll my bed up to the higher level. I was placed with my head facing the heater and the thermostat on my right side at eye level.

I do not have much recollection of that time right after the surgery and who visited me, but I do recall my parents coming quite often. I remember always asking them to raise the temperature higher; for some strange reason, the room seemed a bit cold, and it seemed like I was the first one to use it. Still, I liked the room. It was very private, and the nurses were close by to keep a constant watchful eye on me.

My parents were leaving for the night, they would raise the temperature like I asked them to. Once they left, I closed my eyes until the nurse or my parents arrived the next morning. I remember my dad saying, "Holy cow, it's warm in here," and when they approached my bed, they noticed that my face was red and the blanket was wet, so they lowered the temperature down.

Now the heater blew chilly air toward my bed. When they left for the evening, I closed my eyes, but in the middle of the night I woke up shivering.

I spent a few days in this room, and every night I would have very strange dreams. To this day, I find these nights very confusing. I am not 100% sure which parts were real and which parts were dreams. Some of the dreams are easy to distinguish because they make no sense, but other strange occurrences still feel very real, casting doubt on my sense of reality.

Rape Dreams, Are They?

I was withdrawing $20 bills from an ATM. I put the money in my wallet, but as I turned to leave, I was punched in the face and robbed of the money. I was on the ground screaming for help, but no one showed up. When my attackers had left, I got up, bloody from the assault, and ran inside the bank to call my daughter.

I was resting alone in bed when then the ceiling suddenly started to move. I was being rolled down a hallway that got dimmer and dimmer until there was no visible light. Someone approached and began to touch me in inappropriate places. But then the lights turned on in the hallway, and I started to fight back. I opened my eyes and saw a big steel garage door opening and my parents and my wife coming through it.

Now that my wife was at my side, I was given the choice of her leaving or switching spots with me. I told her to leave, so she did. There were five people by my bedside, and I was unable to defend myself; the only thing I could do was close my eyes until this torture was over. Then I was given a pill to take. I tried to resist, but they forced it into my mouth and made sure I swallowed. I opened my eyes and was in my room with the sunlight on my face.

I was on a platform being rolled into a hallway, turning right, then turning left, then we entered a room where I was stripped of my clothes and sprayed all over with cold water from a hose connected to the wall. I laid naked on the platform, soaked and shivering but unable to speak and too weak to move. I just prayed for it to be over.

I reported this to my wife, who in turn, reported the incident to the head nurse. It was requested that no male nurses be alone with me, and after an investigation it was concluded that the suppository the nurse had inserted while I was asleep might have triggered some of my terrible thoughts.

All these nights were extremely uncomfortable to discuss because my memories were so blurred and confusing. I know I was under a very heavy load of medication which may or may not have played a role in this, but it all felt very real. I honestly think the explanation that was given to my wife was not enough, and many questions remain, but I am glad this is all behind me now.

Hand/PT Development

I spent a few days in my room, then I received a special wooden glove that prevented the fingers on my left hand from curving inward. Whenever I took my hand out of the glove, the fingers on my hand would curl. I wore this glove during all my free time.

After about two days, a new physical therapist came to my room and told me we would start the next day. I was quite depressed at this stage because I had been improving so rapidly in my previous PT, but the last surgery had taken all my gains away and the whole experience now felt like a waste.

In the afternoons, my parents and my wife would come. I do not remember my wife bringing Isabella, but I do remember asking for her. I was extremely disappointed; you could tell from my sad expression and my silence how sad I was that she was never around. I think my parents noticed that I was not quite myself and tried to cheer me up, asking what was bothering me. I told them I wanted to leave the hospital, but the answer was always the same: "You can't right now."

Finally, I was able to get back in my wheelchair and my parents took me downstairs to the lobby. The center of my attention was the cafeteria food. I was thinking how great it would be to eat those French fries. They looked so good, and as I watched people drinking coffee, I was jealous that they could enjoy these things and take them for granted. They seemed to bring the coffee to their lips and swallow it in slow motion, and as I watched them, I could almost taste and smell it for myself.

We went through the lobby and opened the door to an outdoor sitting area. This was in the back middle of the hospital, and they were constructing an additional unit designed for physical therapy patients. We went outside a few times in those days, and what I remember most was seeing the green grass and the tree that grew at the end of the patio about ten meters from the entrance. But anything was better than the inside of my room.

The next morning, the physical therapist entered the room. He was solidly built, with bulging muscles that could be seen through his shirt. He transferred me to the wheelchair with ease and pushed me down the hall to a room on the right side. This was a big room with different PT equipment and a stack of mattresses. I was pushed in front of the mattresses and asked to stand up, using the mattresses for support. I did it, but you could see my wobbly legs looking as if they might buckle at any moment.

I managed two half squats, which was my maximum; after that, I plopped back down in the wheelchair and was pushed toward a table with a few yellow bands tied to the wall.

The physical therapist told me to pull one toward me, so I grabbed the handle of one elastic band with a label that read "10 lbs." *This does not look like hard resistance*, I thought, pulling the elastic band toward my body. I was able to fully pull with both hands three times, and then I was moved over to the mattresses again and told to stand up and without holding onto anything. I was very unsteady; my legs were very wobbly, and I felt as if I would fall if I were not touching anything. I lasted three seconds, then plopped down heavily into my wheelchair with its safety wheels locked on the floor.

As I tried these exercises, it did not occur to me that I had injuries from the surgeries. I did a few reps each day, which lasted about an hour, and each morning I was improving, either by squatting more than on the previous day or by pulling the bands further. Soon I was standing by myself for twelve seconds unassisted, and the feeling of being a young boy was slowly coming back. Standing was my proudest achievement; we did this for a few days until one day the physical therapist said if I was able to pass his "fit test" the next day, I would be transferred to St.

Peter's Hospital in Hamilton, where they specialized in physical therapy and would be able to train me properly.

This information excited me greatly, and when I returned to my room, I did five sit-ups on the bed, lifted the bed sheet until I got tired, then lifted my left leg up until I couldn't lift it any higher, then did the same with my right leg. I felt full of energy and excitement, like a young boy running around after eating a piece of chocolate. Finally, I lifted the pillow until I could no longer lift it, then I repeated everything I had just done. I do not know where this energy came from, but I needed to burn it since I wanted to get transferred so badly.

Looking at the clock above me on the wall, I saw a couple hours had passed. When my parents showed up, I was trying to tell them the news; however, I was gasping for air and sweat was streaming down my face. Some mumble came out of my mouth, but they did not understand what I was saying so I pointed to the letter board, thinking this would be quicker. It seemed to take so long to find that I wanted to explode with the news. Finally, my mom held up the letter board, and I lifted my right arm and opened my pointer finger. *Open faster*, I said to myself. I started to point at the letter G and then at the letter O, my parents started to guess the word, then I pointed to the letter I and they got it—they guessed GOING. I thought to myself, *This is going to take too long*. I pressed the red button to call the nurse. I was so impatient that I pressed it multiple times, and in a few minutes the nurse showed up. She explained what I was doing today, and she told my parents the news that I would be transferred to St. Peter's Hospital if I passed the test the next day. This was extremely exciting for all of us. After an hour, my wife showed up and learned of my possible transfer. We went outside to get some fresh air, passing through the lobby and going outside through the automatic entrance door. We went to our spot and chatted about nothing important, just killing time; however, I did ask for the tempting coffee from the lobby but unfortunately received none. After some time, the moon began to appear in the darkening sky, and we went back to the room. Shortly afterward, my parents left, and my wife and I lay together in bed and watched the Food Network—after all, that was the best channel to watch.

When we could see the streetlights glowing outside, my wife left, and I closed my eyes. Well, at least I tried to close them, but all I could think about was the fit test. I finally passed out from exhaustion, and when I opened my eyes, the first thing I did was a simple stretch. Next, I got into my wheelchair, although I do not remember how I managed this alone.

I pressed the red button on the bed to call the nurse. I wanted to let her know I was ready so she could pass the news on to the physical therapist. She arrived and was surprised to see me in the wheelchair. "Oh, you're in the wheelchair already," she said. I nodded my head up and down. "But it's five in the morning," she said, pointing at the clock in my room. I was a bit confused; it felt like it was way later than 5 a.m. I had never gotten times confused like this before; I must have been so excited that I never bothered to look at the clock above my bed.

The nurse helped me back into bed and left, but I just lay there and admired the ceiling. There was no way I could close my eyes now. I was full of excitement and energy. Nothing would stop me from taking this test. *I must and I will pass this fit test*, I thought to myself. The snowman vision came into my mind, and I felt fully prepared. *Bring it on.*

CHAPTER 12

Fit Test to Leave

I could not stop looking at the clock on the wall, and when 10 a.m. finally arrived, there I was, sitting in the wheelchair. My face might have looked innocent, but inside I was full of excitement for today's test. *It is 10:02 a.m.; he is late!* A hundred thoughts of what could have gone wrong went through my mind, but the physical therapist finally showed up at 10:03 a.m.

"Are you ready for the fit test today?" he asked. I looked up into his eyes and nodded yes. "Super, let's go," he said. He had no idea how important this test was to me, how badly I needed to impress him so he could let me be transferred to St. Peter's Hospital. Getting behind my wheelchair, he started to push me through the hallway to the PT room. I could not shake the smile off my face; I felt reborn, full of energy, ready to tackle any challenge that was thrown toward me. *Here I come.*

We entered the room, and he pushed me in front of a stack of mattresses, asking me to stand up and lean on the top of the mattress for stability. Once I was standing, he asked me to do five half squats. I did seven, looked at him like it had been nothing, and said, "What's next?" He then pushed me over to a machine and instructed me to pull a handle. I grabbed the handle and pulled it toward my body like it weighed nothing. "Good," he said. "Now switch and pull with your left arm." I switched like instructed and again pulled like it was nothing, looking at him and asking, "What's next?" He walked behind my wheelchair and turned me around to face the wall.

Once we got to the wall, he asked me, "Greg, you see those dots on the wall?" I nodded and said yes. He said, "Good. While standing, I want you to touch them three times." I got up from my wheelchair with him right next to me. My heart was hitting my chest, and you could see the sweat on my forehead; I felt my legs wobbling like crazy and found myself thinking I couldn't do this task, but I knew I had to complete my mission. I lifted my right arm and moved it toward the dot, then opened my finger and touched it. In my head was a celebration: *I touched the dot! I did it!* However, when I resumed my original stance, my legs buckled and I plunged hard back to the wheelchair, looking at the physical therapist all confused like, *What just happened?* "Greg, that's enough for today," he said. "I'll take you back to your room."

While he was taking me back to my room, my eyes were watery and inside I was crying harder. I was crying because I knew I was not good enough to be transferred to St. Peter's. Back at my room, he wheeled me over to the window and said he would return later that afternoon. He then left the room, and I let the tears flow, consumed with guilt over my failure. I looked through the window for a good couple of hours until a pigeon landed on the windowsill. "Lucky pigeon," I told it. "Life's so simple for you."

But later that afternoon, the physical therapist came back and said, "Greg, you're going to be transferred to St. Peter's Hospital; you performed better than I expected. Congratulations!" With my heart beating quickly against my chest, I replied, "Really? I thought I failed." "No, no, you performed better than I was expecting. It was a pleasure, and I never met someone that can do so much in so little time. I wish you a quick recovery. Take care; a nurse will give you further instructions," he said, then left. I could not believe what I had just heard. To think I was so worried and jumped to a negative conclusion for nothing. This was super news; *I will not let anyone down*, I thought. *I will recover and build that snowman.* Then my parents came in, and I told them about my transfer at 6 p.m. When my wife showed up thirty minutes later, we shared the exciting news with her, then they all helped me pack up my things and we waited for further instructions.

The nurse showed up and told us that two people would come to take me to the ambulance that would drive me to St. Peter's. Right after she left, the two people showed up and wheeled my bed to the ambulance, telling my parents and my wife where to meet us.

CHAPTER 13

St. Peter's Hospital, About Time

Opening my eyes after the ambulance ride, I saw an elevator and a big sign above it that read *Welcome to St. Peter's Hospital.* They pressed the button to call the elevator and we entered a minute later, the doors closing behind us. I could feel my heart beating quickly in my chest, I was so happy to be there. The elevator started to go up, and I cannot describe all the thoughts that were in my head; however, I do remember the image of my daughter's face. She was throwing a snowball at me, and we were laughing together.

The elevator door opened and as I was slowly moved out, I was getting familiar with my new surroundings. I saw a couple of nurses dressed in blue going into different rooms, and I realized that I would have the opportunity to meet them all. I had already done the impossible, and now I was here to bring energy to this new place. I would surprise everyone and once I left, I would be remembered.

I was moved into my room, and I noticed that mine was the first in the hallway, right next to the nurses' station. The two people who had brought me placed me on the bed and left, and the nurse came in. She hooked up the feeding tube, not for medication but for the liquid food that was to be run 24/7. The plan was to bring my weight up. This bed had a scale, and another nurse came into my room and pressed a button on the bed. I saw my weight for the first time since my admission to the hospital at the same time as she said it: "Greg is 124 pounds." I could not believe I'd lost so much weight. I looked at my arm and noticed the loose skin and the bone that had become visible since I had dropped from my previous weight of 173 pounds.

Food to Fatten Me Up

There were two cans of liquid food hooked up to my feeding tube, with a third can on the top of the desk below and to the right of my bed. From the explanation I intercepted from the nurse, I gathered that more food cans waited below in the cupboard. The nurse informed me that each can would last three hours, and when the cans were empty, the machine would beep until a nurse came to refill it. The machine was to run constantly until they got word from the doctor to adjust the amount of food.

Just then, my parents entered the room along with my wife. Seeing me in bed hooked up to a machine and knowing I'd be there a while, they'd brought me some personal things like my toothbrush, deodorant, cologne, and some pictures of my daughter that they placed on the bedside table next to the Kleenex box. They also brought a couple of magazines for me to read, mostly fitness and some about the brain. We had some time to admire the room, and I was told that I had a roommate but that he was not there just then. It was a nice room, and I was pleasantly surprised to see that it even had a washroom. Out of the three rooms I had been in so far, this was the first to have a washroom. We finished setting up and spent a few hours together in the room. I do not remember having the letter board in that room, but I think it was used once or twice and then taken away since it was too difficult to point at the letters anyway.

After everyone left, I closed my eyes and drifted to sleep. The machine started to beep, but I did not quite wake up and cowered in the darkness. Something I did not know was chasing after me. Then my eyes opened wide and all I could hear was the beep. I pressed the button to call the nurse; the lights turned on, the beep stopped, and I closed my eyes again.

I could hear the nurse replacing the empty cans with full ones and then leaving the room, turning off the light after her. But the rest of the night was horror. Every time I closed my eyes, the machine ran out of liquid food and started to beep. This lasted for a week, then finally I was told that one can would be removed, meaning the machine would only have to run ten hours a day. This was good news; I could finally close my eyes without hearing the beeping.

Roommate

In the morning, I met my roommate, a gentleman in his eighties named James. He could not walk either; I believe he had plunged from a ladder while trimming the branches of a tree on his front lawn and had been in the hospital for a few years. I am not sure how we managed to talk since I was extremely hard to understand, but he did understand my mumble. We chatted a bit and came to know each other very well. James was from British Colombia and had been transferred here because there they did not have all the devices that his condition required. He did not have any family members around since they were all still in BC.

Teaching Me to Eat

My mom always came around lunchtime, and one day she was like, "Why don't we try some home food tomorrow?" I nodded my head yes, thinking it was worth a try.

The next day at lunch, my mom showed up with some thick mixture of different meats. I was very curious what would happen. My mom opened her purse and took out a container with the food, placing it onto my wheelchair tray, then took out the teaspoon and did the same. She opened the container, filled the teaspoon halfway with the food and brought the teaspoon to my mouth. I opened wide, imagining the flavor of food that I missed so much. The teaspoon was in my mouth, and I started to bring my lips together, and boom—the food was now on my tongue. But should I swallow? My head was swimming with thoughts, but the flavor started to drip deeper into my mouth, and I could no longer resist it. I closed my eyes and swallowed. "And? And?" my mom asked. Before I could answer, I started coughing. I coughed for around five minutes, but nothing else happened. I told my mom we should try this again. The same thing happened, but we decided to stop and try again the next day. My mom had to go home but told me she and my dad would come around 6 p.m. She then helped me transfer back into bed and left.

First PT

Later in the day, the assistant physical therapist, Sarah Furgesouin, entered the room and asked me if I was interested in doing some physical therapy. "Of course," I replied. She helped me to transfer into my wheelchair, then pushed the wheelchair into the physical therapy room.

The joy I had in that moment! This was my first time leaving the room, and I took in the life around me—the bustle of the hospital floor, the nurses, and other patients in their wheelchairs. The PT room was just down the hall from my room, and once Sarah pushed me through the double doors, I found myself in an impressive room with a large window and an array of different machinery and beds. Part of the room was carpeted, and her desk was at the end of the room. There were other patients there, and I was parked beside them to await my turn. When my turn arrived, a physical therapist named Sarah Repokel—yes, two Sarahs—approached me. I do not quite remember what we did that day, but I remember feeling my heart beating fast against my chest and my breathing getting rapid after 10 minutes. The assistant therapist, Sarah F., then escorted me back to my room and helped me transfer back into bed. She said she would be back for me the next day at 1 p.m. I nodded my head and said, "Okay, see you tomorrow."

Feeding Practice

The next day during lunch, my mom arrived and wanted to try feeding me again. Once everything was set up, the spoon landed in my mouth again and the new flavors landed on my tongue. Let us not forget here that this was only the second time in weeks that I had experienced the flavors of food in my mouth. I had not even tasted water since being admitted to St. Michael's Hospital. I swallowed the food from my tongue, and a minute later, started to cough, but nowhere near as much as the day before.

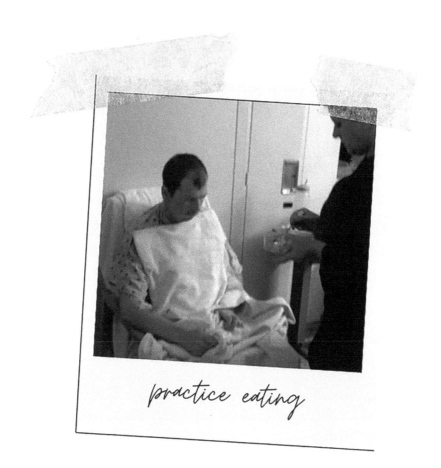

practice eating

Feeling ready to try again, I asked my mom for another spoonful. We both got excited and she piled the teaspoon high with food. She stuck the spoon into my mouth, the food landed on my tongue, and I closed my eyes and swallowed. I waited for the now-familiar cough, but it never came. We looked at each other, puzzled. We waited 15 minutes and nothing—no cough, no nothing—so I wanted to try yet again. This time, I had a gentle cough like my throat was simply readjusting itself. I was not coughing rapidly like I had been. We decided to wait another 20 minutes and tried again, but this time my coughing came back. At this point we stopped, deciding not to push it anymore. "We'll try something new tomorrow," my mom said. She then left, saying she would return later with my dad.

I told the nurses who took care of me about my lunch experience, but their response was not what I wanted to hear. "It's too dangerous; don't do it again." *Why not do it again?* I thought to myself. *It is not harming me, and this feeding by feeding tube is awful; I do not even taste what is injected into my stomach.* I made the decision to continue.

Physical Therapy Again

Sarah F., the assistant therapist, arrived in my room when I saw the sun in the bottom of the window. Eager to go, I was already waiting in my wheelchair. She took me to the physical therapy room, but before I started PT, she placed me in front of a table. A different therapist showed up and we practiced some coordination work and some cutting of dough and placing of toy blocks. After 30 minutes on the huge clock that hung on the wall, she placed me by the other patients waiting their turn for physical therapy.

When it was my turn, I was transferred onto a blue-covered table and asked to do an exercise I had never heard of before: bridging. The therapist instructed to lie on my back, place my feet close to my backside, and lift. I lifted, feeling the stretch in my quads as I used these muscles for the first time. I pushed through the burn but could not do more than three. After bridging, I was told to try lady push-ups, the kind where your knees rest on the table. After two attempts, I was able to do four, after which I was transferred back into my wheelchair, feeling proud of my accomplishment. Then Sarah F. took me back to my room and asked if I wanted to go into my bed. I shook my head no, and she left. I wanted more. I grabbed the pillow off the bed and started to lift the pillow above my head until my face turned red and I was gasping for air. I then placed the pillow back on the bed, satisfied with the day's progress.

Isabella's First Visit

Around 4 p.m., my wife and my daughter Isabella showed up. I immediately felt tears coming to my eyes and my heart pounding against my chest. I didn't want her to be there for too long since my energy level was depleting quickly, and I didn't want her to see me in such a terrible state, but we managed to draw and watch some TV together. It was genuinely nice to spend some time with my daughter and take my thoughts off everything that was happening. They left after 30 minutes, but that time felt like hours to me. Then literally five minutes after they had gone, my parents showed up. I was blessed to be set up in such a way that I was never alone for a long time. I told my parents about my wife and Isabella visiting and we just relaxed.

Trying Coffee When not Allowed

My parents took me downstairs to the lobby and we chatted—well, they chatted—I just nodded my head. I was looking at the coffee cups they were drinking from. I was thinking it would be nice to drink some since I had a major craving for coffee, and I had not had any since my surgeries. My dad was like, "Do you want to try a sip?" I did not know what to say, and it took me a good few minutes to answer. I said, "What the heck, let me try." My dad brought the coffee cup to my lips, and I went into panic mode in my head, thinking *Holy cow, I am going to do this. No going back now.* The cup touched my lips, and I put my right hand around the cup, slowly starting to tilt it upward until the liquid entered my mouth. *Got it, now I need to swallow*, I thought, but I was still panicking. I had been told not to eat or drink, and here I was with coffee in my mouth. My dad was like, "Swallow it! Swallow it!" I looked at him with a frozen, muddled look. *Should I? Should I not swallow?* That was the question in my head at that moment. I closed my eyes and took a deep breath through my nose, and it felt like time was frozen. I started to swallow, feeling as the liquid slowly moved toward the back of my mouth and went down. Looking into my dad's eyes, I told him, "It's done, I swallowed it." But after 20 seconds, I started coughing and coughing like I had never coughed before. My parents started to slap my back, but nothing could stop the coughing. After five minutes of solid coughing, it just stopped, like hitting the brakes in your car. I looked at my parents, very puzzled and with tears in my eyes, and said, "No more coffee today." And we started to laugh. Still, I was happy. "I did it!" I rejoiced. "I drank coffee." The flavor seemed to last for hours. We went outside and chatted some more, and when we started to see stars, they took me back to my room and helped me get into bed.

At first light, I started to get up and transferred into my wheelchair. The first time I attempted this task, it literally took me 30 minutes with breaks in between because I got so tired. I asked the nurse to watch just in case I failed in some way, but I was able to accomplish it without help and she told me I could do this on my own. After numerous attempts, I managed to get into the wheelchair in 10 minutes. Later, around 7 a.m., I called the nurse and told her that I wanted to get washed and changed.

My mom usually arrived at lunchtime, and we attempted to eat home food. I was getting quite a bit better and started to look better from eating what she brought me. By now I was eating hospital food, but let us be honest, hospital food is not very nutritious, nor does it have the best flavor. In the beginning, I struggled to finish everything; after almost every spoonful of food I would have a coughing fit for a few minutes, but when I stopped coughing, we would continue. In the beginning, it took three hours to spoon-feed me a meal, but after a month, this time shortened to two hours, then one hour the next month.

Eventually, I managed to eat by myself, but I still wanted someone to watch me as I was not yet 100% confident in my ability to swallow food of different textures. First this was my mom, then I asked a nurse to stand guard while I ate.

My right arm would shake a bit as I held a utensil, but I managed to finish all the food that was given to me. I got faster and faster until even the nurses were impressed. In bed at Hamilton General Hospital, I had been told by a nutritionist that I would never eat again, but I guess she was wrong.

CHAPTER 14

Speech Therapy

In the morning, a speech therapist named Barbara Zakol came to see me. She started taking me every day about two hours before my physical therapy started. We practiced a variety of phrases, movements, and sounds that could help people more clearly understand what I was saying to them. It turns out that some actors and TV personalities practice speaking this way so they can sound clear on camera. I spent an hour every day with Barbara and soon felt comfortable enough around her to talk more about what was going on in my life. She was nice and I liked being around her, and this helped me to open up in speech therapy.

I told Barbara about my food experience, and she booked me an appointment at McMaster Hospital for a swallowing test. In about a week's time we traveled to the hospital for my test. In the room, an X-ray blanket was placed on my chest, then they turned on the X-ray machine and you could see my insides on a TV screen mounted above. Barbara started by filling a spoon with thick food so we could see what would happen when I tried to swallow it. She put the spoon to my mouth, and I swallowed with confidence, then we all looked at the TV. I saw the food wander down my throat, but the flap in my esophagus never opened; instead, the food went straight into my lungs. We waited for a minute, giving each other puzzled looks. Nothing was happening, but the food had clearly gone into my lungs. Barbara tried again, but this time the flap opened, and the food went into my stomach. I smiled—well, if you call that a smile, more like a half smile—and again nothing happened.

Barbara said, "Okay, let's try thinner food this time." She filled the spoon with thinner food and brought it to my mouth. I opened my mouth, taking the spoon in, then closed my mouth around the food, moved it back with my tongue, and swallowed. We all looked at the TV to see what would happen, but just like before, the food went into my stomach. I looked into Barbara's eyes and said, "I told you nothing would happen." In disbelief, she replied, "Now you're going to try even thinner food," and I said, "Let us do it." I was now greatly confident about this test, thinking this was nothing. *I ate thinner food with my mom, and I even tried coffee. Bring it on.*

She scraped half a spoonful of some thinner food onto the spoon and moved it toward my mouth. I opened my mouth, took the spoon in, then closed my mouth, sucked the food from the spoon, and swallowed it. We then looked at the TV; this time, after 10 seconds, I had a small cough, but this only lasted for five seconds. We decided to go even thinner to see if I could handle it, so Barbara scraped some food that almost resembled liquid onto the spoon. Again, the spoon entered my mouth, and once more I swallowed it. We turned our heads towards the TV to see the food going down my throat; this time, however, the flap did not open. The food entered my lungs—but again, nothing happened. I was not even coughing.

This puzzled everyone who was watching the TV. We waited a few minutes to see how my body would react, and still nothing happened. We decided to go with even thinner food. This time I was less confident of what would happen; I had tried coffee and that had not gone so well, and even though that had been a month ago, I was still skeptical of something this thin. But Barb poured some almost liquid into a cup, let me grip it, and said, "When you're ready." With my eyes on the TV, I moved the cup closer to my mouth, made a small opening, and took a small sip of this stuff. It tasted horrible. Wondering what I would see on the TV, I swallowed. We all watched as the liquid traveled down my throat. It reached the flap, but the flap did not open; the liquid entered my lungs. But I had only a small cough, and even after we waited five minutes, nothing else happened. "Now we're going to try liquid," Barbara declared.

I was even more nervous about liquid, but my success so far made me optimistic. Barbara poured some liquid into a cup, put the cup in my hand, and said once again, "When you're ready." I looked into her eyes and said, "Okay." I moved the cup to my lips, made a small hole, and took a small sip. Among the many thoughts going through my head was an image of me eating steak, but in the end, it was only this foul-tasting liquid that I swallowed. On the TV screen, the liquid seemed to be going down my throat in slow motion. Finally, the liquid reached the flap, which did not open, and entered my lungs. I looked at Barbara, disappointed, and then began to cough. This time, the coughing lasted four minutes. Barbara decided to stop there; we now knew that pure liquid would make me cough and I would need to add a thickening agent to any liquid I wanted to drink. My biggest question of the day was what had happened to the food that entered my lungs?

After the swallowing test we returned to the hospital, and Barbara took me to my room. After we had gossiped for a minute or so, she left.

One memorable morning was when everyone was getting a made-to-order breakfast. After the nurse took my roommate James' order, she asked what I would like to have. Not wanting to complicate things, I just asked for fried eggs. She wrote down the order, but when she came back, only James got a plate of food. I was confused and asked what had gone wrong. She answered, "You can't eat yet," and I replied, "Barbara Zakol, my speech therapist, said I could." The nurse said she would call to check with Barbara and get back to me.

It was a long weekend, so I had no therapy that day. I was in my bed watching the clock tick slowly as the hallway filled with the smell of food. When the clock showed 12 p.m., the nurse returned with eyes wide open. Approaching my bed, she said, "I wasn't able to contact her, I'm sorry," and then left. I felt crushed, having waited all that time only to smell James' food and watch him eat, but at least I could enjoy the meal vicariously through him. The smell in the hallway, which seemed to last for hours, was not helping either.

PT Continued

Before long, I started visiting the physical therapy room by myself. It was not far from my room, so it only took me five minutes to get there. I craved more than the one hour that each patient was assigned and started looking for any chance to rehabilitate my muscles. The constant movement paid off as I began to recover more of my strength.

Sarah R., my therapist, deserves kudos for pushing me to my limits. I had a fun time learning new techniques and developing strength in places where my muscles had gotten weak.

I was disappointed that someone told her I would not be walking and not to waste time on me.

The most memorable moment in PT was when I was put in the middle of a wide red machine. It was like being in a baby's walker where you cannot fall since the walker goes where your body weight goes. So, if you were falling backward, the walker would go backward. In this walker, I made my first attempt at jumping, which I had totally forgotten how to do. After a few attempts, I finally managed a small jump, maybe one inch off the ground. But even better, I could now wander around the hall. Like a bird taking its first flight, I felt proud and free as I walked down the halls by myself, just me and the walker.

Gaining strength felt amazing. I kept getting stronger, and each day I could not wait until my next physical therapy session would begin. I gained so much strength throughout my body that I was able to do 11 knee push-ups. I would like to thank both Sarah's here, especially assistant Sarah F., for putting up with me as I sometimes laughed in her face, and both for their enormous patience with me. Thank you again.

Testing My Touch Response

One afternoon after PT, Sarah R., the physical therapist, showed up in my room and told me to get into bed, where she was going to perform a touch sensation test. I got into bed and she explained that I was to close my eyes and she would either poke me or scratch me in different places on the left side of my body. She took out a needle and began; each time she poked or scratched me, I was to tell her where and what I was feeling.

Sarah poked my knee, and I told her it was my chest; she then proceeded to do a gentle scratch on the bottom of my foot, and I felt a scratch on my upper left leg. Then she touched my left knee, and I guessed correctly. She poked the left side of my cheek, and I was also able to correctly identify this.

She then told me the test was complete and helped me transfer back into the wheelchair. After the transfer, we concluded that my sensation was hugely off, and she left the room.

Refusing the Medicine

As I started to become more conscious of my surroundings, I noticed that several different medications were being injected into my feeding tube, and I wanted to know what exactly I was taking. The nurse explained some of the medications she was giving me, but other medications she could not tell me what they were or what they did. I told her that I gave her permission to proceed with the medications that she'd been able to explain to me, but the ones that hadn't been explained, I refused to take until I knew what they were and what was they were doing. My daily refusal of these meds lasted for around three days until a doctor came—I guess he was a hospital doctor, because I had never seen him before. The doctor explained that one of the medications was for any suicidal thoughts and another was an antidepressant. He said that if I wanted to get off them, I would need to gradually lower my dosage until none was required, since by now my brain would be dependent on the medications. I would be monitored to see how my brain reacted to the smaller dosage and eventual these medications would be removed.

I was a bit alarmed that such medication would be required, but after that explanation from the doctor I allowed the nurse to proceed with the lower dosage as he had explained would need to be done.

I called my wife and my parents to tell them what I had learned and that I was planning to get off of these medications. But when I talked to my wife, I learned that it was she who had given permission for the psychiatric drugs. It had been because of my young age and because they were all afraid of how I would react.

I just wished I had been told this sooner so I could get off it quicker instead of having to refuse it, which I'm sure was awkward for the nurses (although I'm sure they understood my situation).

After two weeks, I was finally off all the medications. Personally, I did not notice any unusual behaviors; my parents noticed that for around a month I was a bit hyper, but nothing too out of the ordinary compared to my normal mood.

Stomach Tube Removal

It was 8 a.m. on a Wednesday morning when the nurse entered my room and told me I needed to be up and ready to go because I was going to Hamilton General Hospital. I asked for further details, but she was not able to tell me anything else, leaving me puzzled. Once I was ready, two gentlemen and a nurse came and moved me into the ambulance for the 15 minute trip. Once we arrived, we entered a room where there were two other nurses. I was placed on the cold table and asked to expose my feeding tube. Finally, my question was answered: I was told they would be removing the feeding tube! This was the most exciting news I had had in days. Visions of various foods entering my mouth and thoughts of different flavors immediately came into my mind. I lay flat on my back on the table and lifted my shirt so they could remove the feeding tube. They started pulling, but the tube seemed to have no end. It took them multiple hand readjustments to finally pull this feeding tube out. Once it was out, I could see that the part that had hung out of my body was clear and the part that had been inside my stomach was dark, but what surprised me most was the length of the feeding tube. The nurses covered the hole with a bandage, and I was then transported back to my room in St. Peter's Hospital.

I was extremely excited that my feeding tube was removed; the second I got to my room, I grabbed the phone, but I struggled to dial the numbers because my hand was shaking so much. All I wanted at that moment was to call and report the news to my family, and nothing was going to stand in my way. I tried calling my wife first, but I kept pressing eight instead of nine; then if I got those numbers correct after multiple attempts, I would press the wrong number in the middle, three instead of two. I tried and I tried, and finally I gave up and called the nurse to dial the number for me. Yes, yes, it was finally ringing…but no one answered at my wife's house. I was disappointed, but I knew I could still call my parents. I called for the nurse once more and she dialed my parents' number and…yes, it was ringing! Now I could finally tell someone the good news!

My mom answered, and I told her in my gibberish speech what had happened, and she understood—well, at least I think she understood, because I remember her saying, "I'll bring cake when I get there, and you're going to eat it on this special day!" She was as excited as I was. After hanging up, I tried calling my wife again. My excitement was tempered now, and I was able to dial the number myself. This time she answered, and I told her the news. In my mind I was already thinking of the steak and wine I would have when I got home. I could almost imagine the juices that would fill my mouth with every bite, and although I knew it would be a while before I could eat steak, I remembered being told I'd never eat again, and I knew every day brought this dream closer to reality. As for my feeding tube, I am not sure how my wife got hold of it, but I was disappointed to learn she had thrown it away without consulting me. I would have liked to keep it to remind me of what I had gone through, and to show our future children this thing that had been in their dad's stomach. But it was gone, and I did not make too much of a stink about it.

CHAPTER 15

Going Home

My wife and I were sitting outside behind the hospital when a strange man approached us. He introduced himself as an eye doctor and said he would like to look at my eye. "Sitting in my wheelchair?" I asked. "Yes, sitting in your wheelchair," he replied and asked my permission to go ahead. Of course, I nodded yes, and he began to examine my eyes. The treatment he decided on was to temporarily shut my right eye by gluing my eyelid hairs together. He took a tube of glue out of his pocket and placed a small dot on my top eyelid hairs, then lowered my top eyelid, pushed it together with the bottom eyelid, and held them together for a minute. With that, my right eye was shut, and the eye doctor left.

I had my right eye shut for about a week, and when it fully opened back up, my double vision had disappeared temporally and I was able to see normally—well, at least I thought my vision was normal until I tried reading a magazine and the letters seemed fuzzy. But I did not mind the fuzziness so much, and after looking at the pictures, I put the magazine away.

The next day, I left 30 minutes early for PT because I wanted to check my email on the computer in the lobby. Once seated at the computer, I clicked on the internet browser, but the text on the monitor seemed blurry. Ignoring this fact, I typed my destination in the address bar, but when I finally logged into my email, it was too blurry to read the emails or see who they were from. This really frustrated me, so I brought my face closer to the monitor until my nose was three inches from the screen, and I could finally make out the text. Once I had read everything, I wanted to read the news, but by now my hand holding the mouse was shaking. *Forget it,* I thought, *I do not have the time for this.* With that, I left for my physical therapy.

Trying Electric Stimulation

Since I had no feeling on my left side, the physical therapist tried placing a pad on my left arm before my workouts which would give some electric stimulation to contract and release the muscles and try to restore equal strength to my left arm. I did this for around 10 minutes for a few days in a row, but I did not notice any difference in my left arm strength. It did, however, teach me to distinguish the different strengths in my limbs. I began to work out each limb on its own so I could notice its strong points and weak points and adjust for that limb to have the same strength as the other limb.

An Embarrassing Moment

My wife arrived that afternoon and we went outside, but as soon as we got onto our usual path, I told her I needed to pee right away. She reminded me that I had a diaper on and said to just go, and although I am sure I had used it before, this was the first time I was aware of using it. I took a moment to think, but then relieved myself. I must say this was awkward and I was unsure how to react. I remember peeing my pants when I was eight years old, crying and running to the house, but this was different; I was grown and no longer a kid.

After a moment of shock, I tried to accept what had just happened, and we continued our walk. But as my wife pushed my wheelchair along, I still could not believe what I had done. It stayed in my head the entire day. Through the numerous conversations I had that day, the peeing was always a silent thought that stuck in my mind. I could not really discuss this with my wife; I was still in somewhat of a state of shock, and when she asked about it, I was silent, like a child holding a secret.

After spending about two hours outside, we went back to the room, and I called the nurse to change my diaper with a fresh one. This was the most embarrassing part of the day. I know nurses deal with this on a regular basis, but it was an experience I would not soon forget, and I feel strange sharing this experience with you even now.

Diaper Removal Finally

Some time passed, and I decided to finally be free of this diaper. I knew when I had to relieve myself, and I was able to hold it if necessary. I took it off when I was getting dressed in bed in the morning, and I must say what a feeling of freedom it was. No longer did I have this big bulge in my backside; now I could move freely, with all the space in the world and nothing pressing into me.

I started going everywhere without wearing the diaper—outside to my physical therapy, to my speech therapist, and most importantly, to my room. I had to share how different this new way of moving felt, so I called my wife and parents to tell them of my diaper decision. I told them that it had been making me extremely uncomfortable; after all, I was grown up and this was just weighing me down. Of course, they supported my decision, and I never put on a diaper again.

Weekends at Home

Since I was doing extremely well in my recovery, I was now allowed to go home for the weekends. This was extremely good news. My wife would pick me up around 4 p.m. on Friday and return me on Sunday evening. It was nice to get a change of scenery and to see faces besides the ones I always saw in the hospital.

But when I asked about Isabella, my wife told me she was at her parents' house. I left it at that, not wanting to start a fight, but it seemed she was never around on the weekends. In my head I wondered why, during the only time I had to spend with her, she was always at my in-laws.

I'll never forget one weekend when I was finishing up in the washroom and called my wife for help leaving. When we reached the hallway, she kicked my leg. I said, "What the heck are you doing?" She told me she was trying to get me to walk straighter. This did extreme emotional damage, leaving a scar like a name engraved into a tree. But I pretended nothing had happened and flopped down on the couch when we got to the living room.

Chess With Dad

Sometimes when my mom could not visit, my dad came. We usually went through the lobby and out onto the patio beside the hospital. We grabbed a spot at a table and my dad sat down, pushing me to a space across from him so we could play a round of chess. It was extremely difficult for me to grab and move just one piece with my shaking hand; often I would knock over other pieces in the process. But it was a good coordination exercise, and we enjoyed the games; a round usually lasted a few hours.

Out of St. Peter's Hospital and Extremely Excited

Finally, after six months at St. Peter's Hospital, I was released to go home for good. That day felt so good. My mom bought a box of donuts and a coffee for everyone, but unfortunately these were not for me—I still could not swallow liquids and eating often still provoked coughing fits. But nothing could take away my excitement to leave the hospital. I packed and got ready to go; my mom and I waited for my wife to arrive, and when she finally did, they helped me into our car, and we drove home. I could not wait to finally spend some time with Isabella.

We arrived at the house and went inside, but it was empty. No Isabella, nobody to welcome me back. I must say I was extremely disappointed in that moment. In the back of the house was my father-in-law working on a fence post. We said hi to one another, and then he resumed his work like nothing had happened, dealing me another emotional blow on my big day.

The next day, my dad brought over a handrail that he had built as well as a heavy blue walker for me to practice walking in. Without help, however, I was extremely limited in what I could do. My wife's work insurance would cover five sessions of physical therapy, so I started going to a place that was only 15 minutes from our house. But because I was taking a paratransit bus that picked up many other people on the way there, the trip took an hour and a half each way.

Unfortunately, this physical therapy clinic was a big waste of my time and I did not learn anything there. When I came back from my first PT appointment, I wheeled myself up the small ramp to our front door and tried to put my key in the lock. This was not an easy task, especially in a wheelchair that kept rolling backward. Just when I had finally gotten the key in place however, I rolled back and fell off my wheelchair, tipping it over on its side. I broke down in tears, not because I was hurt, but I felt so alone and normal life seemed so far away. After I had pulled myself up, I promised myself this would change, and I would do whatever I could to recover fully.

Planning a Trip for Adult Stem Cells

After extensive research, I decided to have an adult stem cell procedure on January 16, 2010. The idea was that the stem cells would repair the damaged area of my brain and restore my balance. As this procedure was not available in North America, I booked a flight to Cologne, Germany. This was an awfully expensive procedure, and as we were living off one income, it put a huge strain on our finances. Of course, we borrowed a lot of money, but it wasn't enough, and I decided to swallow my pride and ask for help.

I was to leave after New Year's and my mom would fly with me to Poland; the next day, I would fly to Germany and meet my wife for the stem cell treatment, then she would return to Canada and I would fly to Poland to stay for a while and do physical therapy, since it was way cheaper there than in North America.

CHAPTER 16

Unexpected Help

I got an email from my friend, Ursula Köster Páez, who had left the country years before to reunite with her extended family. We had kept in touch, and I had told her about my situation around the time of my first surgery. The email said that Ursula had sent something for me to her parents' house. I let my wife know, and we drove the 20 minutes to the house where Ursula used to live, and where her parents still lived. Once we reached their house, my wife knocked on the door and Ursula's dad answered. He told my wife to wait, that they had something for us, and when he returned, he gave my wife a package, then he and Ursula's mom came down to the car to greet me. We chatted with them for a couple minutes, then drove back home. Once home, we sat down on the couch with the package between us and started to rip into the wrapping paper.

I could not believe my eyes—there was a pink blanket and some cute clothing for Isabella and some funds that Ursula and her loving family had sent to help with my treatment. Tears came to my eyes instantly, and I raised my head to look at my wife with a feeling of redness in my face. I was in disbelief over this gift and could not make any words come out, but my silent expression told it all.

The next day, I got an email from Ursula's extended family, who live in Germany. They offered us a place to stay until my treatment was complete. Again, I was in disbelief. No one had done something like this for me before. I would understand such a gesture from family (although this never happened either) but from people who had never met me? I was speechless; this act of kindness touched me deeply and would never be forgotten.

Thank You

My former co-worker, Vlad Spehar, did an amazing job organizing a fundraiser for my procedure, and I would also like to thank Bonnie Feeney for her support; it would not have been possible without her. Thank you.

To my surprise and joy, everyone at my former company pitched in, and I was thrilled by the amount of support I received. Thank you to everyone who made this journey possible.

Hotel in Germany

Once we arrived in Germany, we took a taxi the six blocks from the airport to our hotel. Luckily, the taxi driver spoke English. We entered the hotel through a set of big brown doors engraved all over with images of different buildings, proceeded straight through the hallway, and checked into our room. It was on the second floor and quite basic with a bed, a big window, and a washroom and shower, but on the lower level there was a swimming pool which we got into once. It also had a room off the lobby with buffet-style appetizers for when we got hungry during the day.

The Treatment in Germany: Adult Stem Cells

After getting settled in, we left the hotel and took a taxi, not realizing our destination was only three blocks away. We were dropped off in front of the building and entered through the automatic door. To the left were some paintings hanging on a brown wall, and to the right was a couch and the elevator. We proceeded to the elevator and pressed the button for the second floor, where a label said where the clinic was located.

The elevator stopped on the second floor and we got out, walking through the hallway to the reception desk to tell the receptionist we had arrived. She told us to take a seat and wait until we were called. When the doctor came and called us, we entered his office, and I was told to move myself onto the bed and lift my shirt. The doctor poked a needle into my lower back and removed some spinal fluid. After that was done, I was transported into a different office where they poked a needle into the back of my pelvic bone and removed some bone marrow. I was then told to come back the next day for the procedure, when they would insert the stem cells back into my spinal fluid, going to my brain. These tests had only lasted for maybe 20 minutes, and afterward we went back to the hotel.

The next day arrived, and this time my wife pushed my wheelchair the three blocks to the clinic. I could feel a gentle wind on my face and see the shadow of the wheelchair on the grass. After a block or two, the pavement changed; I could feel the bumps through the wheels of my wheelchair. Finally, we reached the clinic. The automatic door opened and we went inside, passing six people on our way to the second floor. Millions of thoughts were going through my head as we waited for the elevator, then went inside and the doors slid closed. We pressed the second-floor button, and we started to move. My legs began to twitch side-to-side, and I began to fidget. The door opened and we entered the hallway. As we traveled through the hallway toward the receptionist, we passed people from all over the world who had come there to have this procedure done. We informed the receptionist of our arrival, and she told us to sit down on the couch that was against the wall.

The doctor entered the room with a syringe and told me that it contained 18 million stem cells with a 92% vitality rate and a 40% success rate. The procedure could take one to three months to be effective. I was transferred onto the bed, lying on my stomach. The doctor lifted my T-shirt, exposing my back, then counted the vertebrae and the spaces in between the bones where the spinal fluid flows. He then injected the liquid that contained my stem cells, and we waited ten minutes. I experienced no pain, but he gave me some pain medication just in case, and we went back to the hotel. The next day, I had minor back pain but dealt with it. It was not until the third day that the real pain of the procedure kicked in. I could no longer sit, lie down, or move; everything I did was painful. The pain meds did not do their job, and I got high from taking so many. After the sixth day, the pain finally went away.

Flight to Poland

When my wife dropped me off at the airport departure lounge, the person sitting across from me with headphones in his ears looked at me and smiled. I did not know how to react, so I just moved to a different spot to wait until I was called. After I had waited for half an hour, a person dressed in a black suit called my name. I raised my hand to identify myself, and he came and pushed my wheelchair onto the plane. As I was being pushed, the waiting passengers looked at me as if I had something stuck to my back.

I was the first to board the plane and was seated by the window. Once everyone was seated, the airplane started to move. Through the small window, I could see the lights of Cologne. The airplane lifted off the ground, and the buildings got smaller the higher the plane went.

As we crossed the air border into Poland, the weather changed to a blizzard, and all I could see through the window was falling snow. Then the cabin lights turned on, and I could no longer see snow, only my reflection. After flying for 40 minutes, I saw a set of small lights. A few minutes later, I saw the same lights, but bigger. Finally, I could see an airport. *This must be where we are landing.* Yes, we were landing there; we were flying in circles and getting closer with each one. Now I could see cars, and the airplane was still going lower. I felt the runway as the plane touched the ground. The plane started to brake once it had slowed down and moved toward the terminal. When I was the last one left on the plane, three people escorted me toward the exit door. They helped me get into my wheelchair, then carried the wheelchair with me in it down the stairs to the tarmac. Inside the airport, I was reunited with my mom, who had gotten there earlier.

Reaching Poland

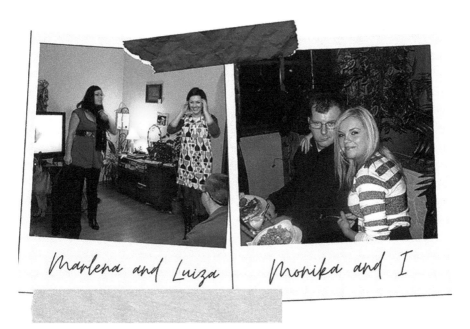

Marlena and Luiza | Monika and I

Once I arrived in Poland, my mom and I stayed with my uncle, Pawel Stołek, and his wife, Basia. We were greeted by their daughters, Marlena and Luiza, along with their cousin, Monika, and over the next few weeks they took me to visit several places I had not seen since my childhood. It was nice to see how the city had changed over the years from what I remembered, to see the apartment building where I'd grown up, which, like many of the apartment buildings, had been painted bright new colors.

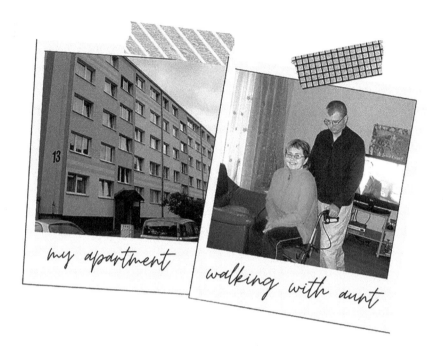

my apartment

walking with aunt

The church was the same as I remember, but the nearby park where I used to play tag had been expanded, and with my limited eyesight I could no longer see the brick school through the trees. Sometimes my uncle would drive my mom and I to the physical therapy clinic, and we would stop on the side of the road to take in the surroundings. I would sit outside the car in my wheelchair and just breathe deeply. I could taste the snow-covered mountains when I took a deep breath, and sometimes we could see smoke drifting up from a chimney far away in the mountains. It was totally different scenery than what I was used to.

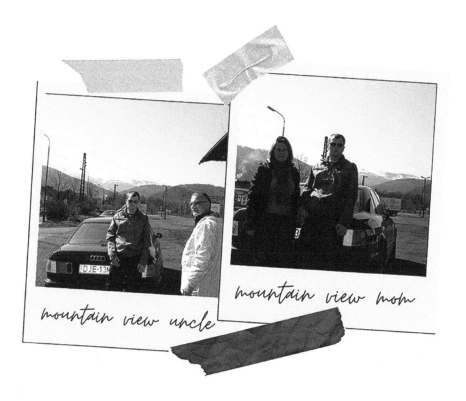

mountain view uncle

mountain view mom

Cousin Surprise

One day while I sat at the kitchen table, someone walked up behind me and covered my eyes with their hands. A voice started whispering in my ear; it sounded familiar, but I still was not certain who it was. But then the person uncovered my eyes, and I instantly recognized her. She looked a little older, but I could never forget those blue eyes and that smile. Tears came unbidden to my eyes. I could not believe it—it was Kasia Siofer, the cousin I had always been closest with.

Kasia would visit whenever she had free time, and we would chat a bit to take our minds off everything that was going on in both of our lives. The last time we had seen one another was in 1989, and it was great to see her and catch up on all the gossip I had been missing.

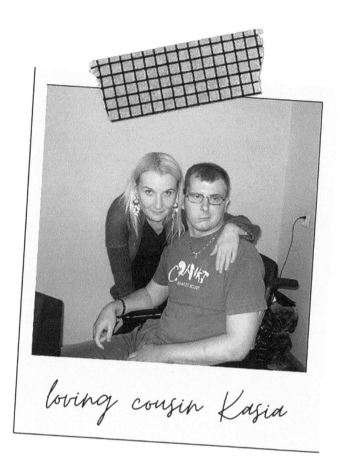

loving cousin Kasia

CHAPTER 17

Physical Therapy in Poland

In the mornings, I went to PT. The doctor who organized all the patients' training was named Dr. Milko, and after I had discussed my situation with him, it was decided that I would get the best results by training with him personally. When he was busy, I would be trained by one of his staff until he could get back to me.

I learned a lot about physical therapy from Dr. Milko, who pushed me to my limits. I remember strolling with him on my knees across the whole room, which was about 50 meters long and had mattresses covering the floor. On the back wall were Swedish ladders where I practiced my balance by sitting on a ball.

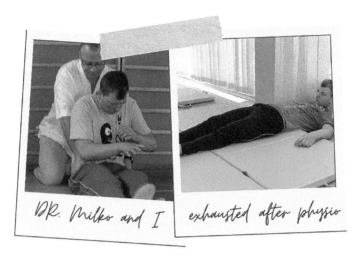

DR. Milko and I | exhausted after physio

The first time I tried rolling across the room, my heart was pounding fast in my chest, and I was breathing rapidly. Dr. Milko approached, and in an encouraging tone, he told me to move onto my knees. He knelt in front of me, grabbed onto my warm arms, and told me to finish the journey to the other side of the room on my knees.

At that point traveling so far on my knees seemed almost impossible, but we began. I lifted my right knee and put it down two inches in front of my left, then shifted my weight onto my right knee where I felt comfortable. Then I lifted my left knee to match my right and held it steady. I had done it, but I was feeling the burn in my quads. By the time I reached the other side of the room, sweat was pouring down my face and I thought I was finished for the day, but I was wrong. Dr. Milko said, "Good, good, now we do it the whole way backward." My quads were on fire, but I knew it had to be done so I ignored the burn and we started, my heart pounding like crazy against my chest. I only managed to make it a third of the way across the room before plummeting from exhaustion. I lay there on the mattress like a fish gasping for air for around 10 minutes before my mom was called to assist me in getting back into the wheelchair. I had never felt so tired before. I was red all over and my shirt was completely soaked. It was the first time I had learned how to move on my knees and how to roll my body, and it would continue to be tough for the first few weeks, especially rolling to the left. Sometimes Dr. Milko's wife, Małgosia, trained me, and she pushed me to my limits as well. This was real training that I knew would bring results—nothing compared with the physical therapy I had experienced before.

Since the Milko's and I spent so much time together, we became close acquaintances and we keep in touch to this day. I will never forget the knowledge I gained of physical therapy, so different from what was done in Canada, and I know they will never forget me. Thank you.

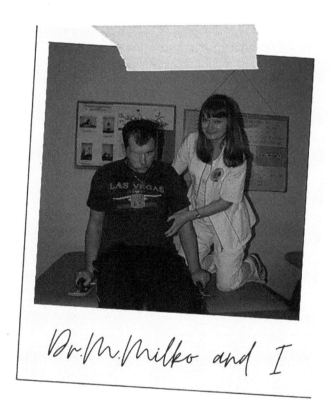

Dr. M. Milko and I

Right Eye in Trouble

One day I noticed a black tear drop out of my right eye and onto my pants. I had been prescribed an antibiotic cream to put into my eye, and I knew something was wrong. I instantly called my mom, but it was too late in the afternoon to visit the eye clinic that day, so she said she would take me the next morning.

The clinic was in some sort of private residence; pine and spruce trees lined the pleasant path that led up to the front door. We went inside and straight to the lobby to check in with the secretary, who told us to wait in the lobby and that the doctor would call us when he was ready.

We took our seat on chairs in the lobby and waited to be called. There were only three people ahead of us, so it was not long before the secretary called us into the doctor's office and sat me in the chair with the weird but familiar machinery at eye level. The doctor came in after us, sitting in front of me and adjusting the machine to meet my eyes. He then looked into the machine, which was pointed at my right eye, and exclaimed, "Oh my God, why haven't you come earlier?" He said he would try to save my right eye using a slew of medications, and that if they didn't bring any improvement, I should report to the hospital, meaning I would lose my right eye. The doctor dropped a couple drops of medication into my eye, then gave us four prescriptions that we had to get filled in the next two hours before the drops stopped working. We succeeded, visiting four different pharmacies to buy the four different medications.

I remember my mom giving me eye drops every few hours, but we saw improvement and reported back to the eye clinic in a few days as instructed. The eye doctor looked at my eye and agreed that it was much improved. He concluded that the antibiotic I had been using before had been used too often and the bacteria had become resistant to it. Since I had paralysis on the right side of my face, which was preventing me from blinking to clear any debris, the doctor suggested inserting a gold plate in my right eyelid to add some weight to it and help me blink. He assured me I would not even notice it was there. I agreed and the procedure was booked.

When we arrived at the building my procedure was to take place in, I saw that it was incredibly old and must have belonged to a lord. It was yellowish in color and had huge floor-to-ceiling windows double the height of a door and statues of knights on horseback with swords and shields flanking the steps up to the door. Between each pair of windows were smaller statues of knights on foot, also holding swords. I was extremely impressed by the outside of the building, but inside it was even more breathtaking. We went in through a huge entrance and saw a grand stairway leading up with a red carpet in the middle and a big sparkly chandelier hanging from the two-story ceiling. We were met in the hallway by one of the surgeon's staff, who guided us down a long hallway lined with doors to different rooms. After walking for a minute, we turned and entered a room on our right. We were met by the doctor and three more of his staff who would be assisting him with the procedure. I was transferred into a chair, which then turned flat, and given several injections. One needle was poked into my right eyelid to numb any feeling or sensation I might have.

Two minutes after I was given the anesthetic, the procedure began. I remember seeing the scalpel that was slowly cutting my eyelid, but I did not feel pain, only the pressure of the cutting and the slow opening of my eyelid. When the incision was finally made, the surgeon asked for the box with the gold plate — I had been told it weighed 2.5 grams. He opened the box, took out the plate, and inserted it into my eyelid. Once it was secure, he started to sew my eyelid back together. I remember trying to squint my eyelid halfway to make it easier for him to sew it together, although I am not sure if that helped because I could not feel if my eyelid was moving. Finally, the surgeon finished. I was relieved; holding my eyelid half-open for 20 minutes proved more difficult than I could have foreseen. The doctor then closed my eyelid and covered my right eye with bandages. He told me to leave them on for two weeks and then to report to him for a checkup.

I was done. The whole procedure had lasted no more than one hour, but to me it felt like it had been several. We were free to leave, and we drove back to Pawel Stołek's house.

After two weeks, we reported back to the doctor, who removed the bandages from my right eye and confirmed that everything was healing correctly.

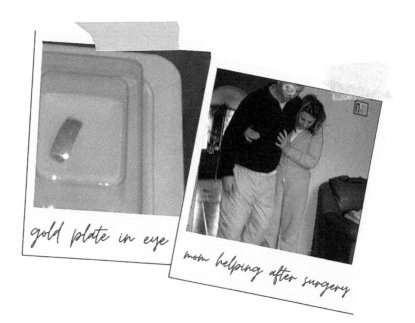

gold plate in eye

mom helping after surgery

CHAPTER 18

Separation via MSN Messenger Chat, Really?

My mom and I stood at an ATM as a line formed behind us. We were trying to withdraw the funds I would need to pay for the eye surgery, and it had failed to authenticate the first time. Figuring I had put in my PIN wrong, I tried again; however, the same thing happened. I felt my face go red and heat spread over my body. I tried putting in my PIN once more, but again it would not authenticate, and we left in confusion.

I contacted my wife over internet chat and told her what had happened. She said she was getting a separation—a requirement to apply for divorce in Ontario—and had everything blocked but would not tell me the reason. I could not believe she could do this to me while I was in a different country, to terminate all their financial assets and leave them on their own. She had also spread false information to my friends and family, and she could have known that all of this would give me tremendous difficulty in my situation. Luckily, I was with my mom and loving friends who were able to provide essential financial and emotional support.

Visiting Mom's Place

Before we returned to Canada, my mom wanted to visit her parents' house. As we neared their house, the first thing that greeted us was the smell of freshly baked bread. Then my mom's father, Bronislaw Kaszczuk, her brother Piotr, and several other family members came out to greet us along with a fresh round loaf of bread. We stayed with them for about a week, and sometimes my mom and I would take walks around the neighborhood, me learning to use a walker and Piotr helping by making sure the path was clear. My mom's family has chickens, and this was also my first time holding a chicken and first time waking up to a rooster crowing.

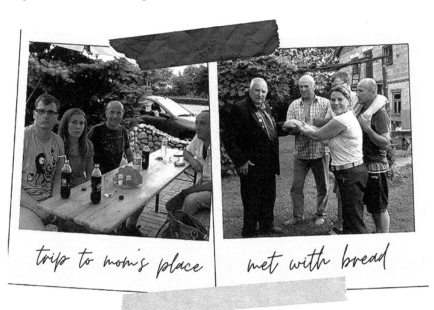

trip to mom's place   met with bread

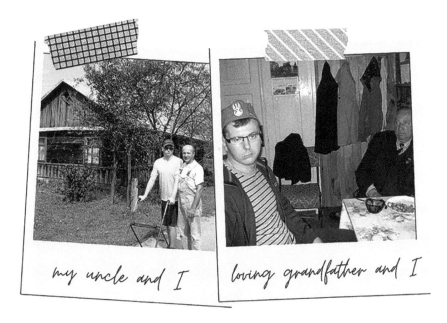

my uncle and I   loving grandfather and I

Returning to Canada From Poland

After eight months in Poland, I went back to Canada. Since my wife had broken up with me over internet chat when I was in Poland, I went to live with my parents. I was still in disbelief that someone could make such a horrendous emotional attack on someone who was very vulnerable and in another country. Even now, she continues to be exceedingly difficult and every interaction with her is an uphill battle.

But I wanted to impress my dad when I arrived in Canada. I wanted his first sight of me in the arrivals section of the airport to be me strolling independently with a walker. Unfortunately, this was not the case; I was still in a wheelchair. However, I was stronger and more active than my dad remembered, so at least he could tell that something had changed. We arrived at my parents' house—my dad had driven his truck, knowing that all our luggage wouldn't fit in a car—and I got out of the truck, leaned on the door, and asked my dad to get the walker. Now was the time to show my improvement. He brought the walker, and I grabbed the handles and positioned myself to walk, leaning slightly forward as I had been trained to do in Poland so that my weight was partially on the walker. I started to move one foot, then the other, then again one foot, then another —*Yes, I am doing it*! Just like I had been taught. I lifted my left foot to take another step, but then I started to wobble. My dad caught me in time, preventing me from plunging, but I wanted to cry just then; I had wanted so badly to show my improvement, and it was devastating to fail.

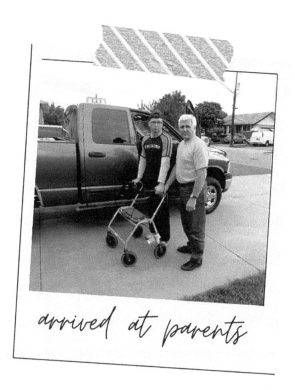

arrived at parents

Later in the day, I was taking a bath, and I gripped a pole on the left side of the bathtub to pull myself up and out. On my way up, I slipped, plummeting straight down onto the floor with a sound that could be heard across the house.

My dad came up to check on me, and at that moment, my eyes began to tear up. I told him I had been trying to get a new towel since mine was a bit wet, and I could not even reach the towel rack beside the sink without falling. My emotions just exploded, and I had tears in my eyes and was mumbling stuff that no one understood. I really broke down; it was just overwhelming with everything that was happening to me. We looked into each other's eyes and his were wet, too. For a few minutes, he just held me. He then helped me go downstairs, and I flopped down on the couch and turned on the TV. After a couple minutes, my emotions settled down, and I went back to normal.

The next morning, I sat at the kitchen table and opened my laptop, beginning to search for exercises to learn how to walk. A couple hours of research proved fruitless, but I did the exercises I had learned from previous research and began to target the areas that needed to be developed. I subscribed to a couple magazines and my friends bought me some books with various exercises. I wanted to continue the things I had learned as well as expand my knowledge by making small adjustments to the exercises I found in my research.

If I found an exercise in a magazine, I usually ripped out the page and made notes on how I would modify it. If I found an exercise while searching online, I would print out the article, and if it was from a book, I would either dog-ear the page or just rip it out.

I read numerous articles about nerve function, the brain, and physical therapy. I also found myself wanting to modify the exercises I had learned from PT in Poland. I had a feeling they could be improved, and a question began to surface often in my mind: *How can a person teach you things they have never gone through themselves?*

I had kept up with all the exercises I had been taught, but my progress seemed to have stalled. This puzzled me deeply. I had read articles on this subject that told me, like the doctors had, that I would not be able to walk again. But I had already proven the doctors wrong, and I knew I would find a way to prove these articles wrong. too.

So, I adjusted and focused on the parts of my body that I saw needed improvement and slowly I began to improve. This confirmed my suspicion that many of the articles I had read were wrong. Again, I wondered, *How you can write an article about relearning to walk if you have never relearned to walk?*

Acupuncture Hype Crushed

One day while browsing through articles, I stumbled on one about the potential of acupuncture to stimulate different nerve endings. This grabbed my attention, and I wanted to see what acupuncture could do in my situation. We decided to meet with an acupuncturist so I could see if it would work as well as I had been told it would.

My first visit, he laid me down on the table and stuck tiny needles in me, first on my face, then on my back. I did not experience any pain, but I saw and felt my leg muscles twitching as if for no reason. The second time, after he placed the needles in my body, he connected some of them to a machine that released an electric current for 15 minutes. As my appointments continued, he would sometimes come to my parents' place to perform the acupuncture since it was quicker to get me ready.

I went through acupuncture for about two months, but I did not notice any difference in my situation and decided to stop.

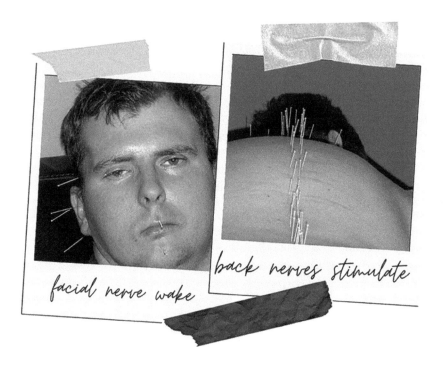

facial nerve wake

back nerves stimulate

A Friend

One day when I was seated at the kitchen table, the phone rang. My mom answered and said it was for me. It was my old co-worker, Connie DeChaves, wondering about my progress. It was great to hear from her, and we chatted about my situation and my future. Not everyone calls to see how you are doing, so this was a nice surprise. We keep in touch on an occasional basis, and I consider Connie the grandmother I never had here in Canada.

BrainPort on Trial

Another day as I looked through a magazine, a device called BrainPort caught my attention. I investigated this device further and found out that it helps you recover balance using your tongue. I was impressed with the reviews and the numerous customer success stories, so I decided it was worth a try.

After visiting a physical therapy clinic, I was able to acquire the device and get instructions on how to use it. I was full of excitement that this might help restore my balance. As soon as we got home, I tore off the packaging and my mom hung the device around my neck and helped me stand (I had to turn on the device in a standing position so it would know the proper alignment). I then placed a small sensor on my tongue which was connected to the device.

I switched on the device and tried standing like I had been told, ready to recover my balance. After trying this for about two weeks, I started to question it since I had not noticed any difference, but I did not give up; I stayed strong and motivated. But after another week had passed, I started to feel disappointment, like a child who has had a toy taken away. I took off the machine, flopped back down on the chair that I used to help me stand, and in a broken voice called my mom to bring the package for the device. Heavy with disappointment that the highly praised device had not worked for me, we packed up the BrainPort and sent it back.

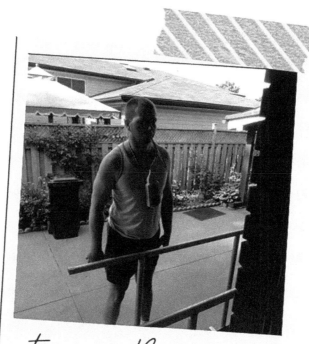

trying Brainport

CHAPTER 19

Back to Hamilton General

A couple days later, we got a call from Dr. Oczkowski's office to come in for a check-up. He was my neurologist, and after we discussed my progress in physical therapy, I was readmitted to Hamilton General Hospital to resume PT there. They had just finished construction on a physical therapy department exclusively for patients with mobility issues, and I was excited to see it, but especially to experience the swimming pool they had built for physical therapy.

I personally did not care too much for the physical therapy, although it did give me the idea to get a treadmill later. Pool therapy, however, was a new experience, and I was ecstatic. After just a couple days of normal physical therapy, the therapist finally told me that for further development, I would be starting swimming pool therapy the next day.

Trying Pool PT in the Hospital

I had read articles about pool PT, but no article can compare to the real thing, and I was beyond excited to start. The next day, my mom and I arrived at the pool therapy department, and I was transferred from my wheelchair onto the platform that lowers you into the swimming pool.

The physical therapist was in the pool in front of me, and the platform started to lower. I felt the warm water lap against my feet and watched as my legs were slowly submerged. The water slowly came higher, and now my shorts were underwater. When the water had reached my belly button, the platform stopped, and the safety rail was opened. The physical therapist instructed me to slide into the water, so I put my hands on the platform at my sides, raising myself slowly and gently pushing forward until I could not go any further and started sliding. With my right hand, I gripped one of the pipes that were used as holds, then slowly let my body slide down into the pool. I had done it; I was in the pool. Now I could feel the warm water reaching my chest.

The therapist told me to begin walking toward the right side of the wall. I noticed the swimming pool had different levels, like platforms, and that you had the option of going lower or higher; I was going lower. Soon the water was touching the top of my chest, and for the first time since the surgery, I was standing fully on my own two legs. I held on to another pipe with my left hand and, with small steps, began to walk toward where the physical therapist was waiting. I was feeling good—incredibly good and incredibly happy. We did a few different exercises, and unlike in outside physical therapy, I could feel my balance improving dramatically and quickly.

I continued pool therapy for three more weeks, and since I was continuing to make so much progress, I was surprised when I was abruptly told it was over. Not ready to stop, my mom and I started going to a recreation center that had a swimming pool with warm water. At first, I wore a life jacket in case I went underwater, but after just a couple of days, despite my mom's nervousness, I stopped wearing it. I was improving very quickly, and after only two months, I could move across the pool without losing my balance and plunging into the water. One benefit of working on my own rather than with a physical therapist was that I could increase the difficulty and push my limits; my mom and I could try whatever we wanted without being told it was too dangerous. I surprised even myself with some of the things I was able to do, and no doubt this freedom was why I was improving so much faster. Sometimes my dad would join us, and I would be able to try even more challenging exercises; my mom was afraid she wouldn't be able to catch me if I fell, so I would practice the more extreme exercises with my dad and then continue them with my mom once I had improved enough to make us comfortable.

Surprise Treadmill for Training

Back at home one day, we heard knocking and my dad went to answer the door. I had an unexpected visitor: my friend, Stefanie Biggar, delivering a treadmill for my training. I did remember mentioning something to her about looking for one since I had seen an exercise that might be effective in training me to walk, but I was shocked when she showed up at my door with one. I could not believe she would do this for my recovery, and it reminded me that there are people out there with warm hearts. I quickly asked my mom to get some coffee brewing and to get the cake she had baked earlier. With tears in my eyes, I hugged Stefanie and thanked her for this unexpected and thoughtful gift. I will always remember this gesture, which touched me deeply. I was lost for words, and all I could say was thank you.

My dad built a strap to attach a safety harness just above the treadmill to prevent me from falling, and I got started. I was pleasantly surprised with my progress; in the beginning, I was extremely nervous and tired quickly, only managing one minute before turning red like a lobster, but after a couple months, I could walk on it for an hour, sometimes with a two-minute break in the middle and sometimes with no break at all. I still use the treadmill all the time since it closely resembles walking—although my walks are much longer today.

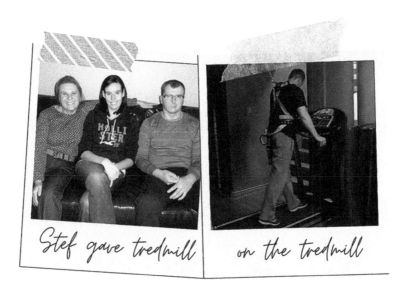

Stef gave tredmill *on the tredmill*

*Isabella's First Communion —
I Thought We Were Adults?*

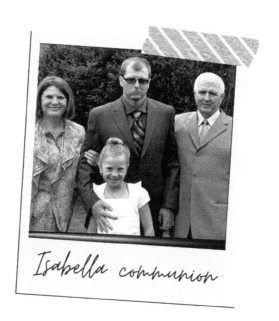

Isabella communion

A few weeks later was my daughter's first communion, so I dressed in black pants and a purple shirt, and my dad drove me to the church with the green walker in the trunk of the car. We arrived at the church, and I began to stroll up the ramp to the left side of the church door, my mom beside me holding onto me and the walker. My daughter saw me and came running toward me, hugging both of us and then leading us to our seats. We opened the door to the church and made our way down the red-carpeted floor to the second row of pews. I squeezed in sideways and sat down in the middle of the pew. On my left sat my family, and my ex-wife and her parents were seated on my right. If only the priest knew of her sins, things might have gone differently. After the communion ended, we were in front of the church where my ex-family members were taking pictures and my friend, Robert Lasinski, nudged me to look across the street. I followed his gaze and saw my grandfather on my dad's side watching us from a distance—just like in a comedy movie, staring but cowardly avoiding any contact. I am not surprised I received zero support from them, and I would have been too embarrassed to anyway. But then my daughter came over to us, and we were able to take a couple of pictures. After the pictures, my parents and I walked away, not invited to the party that would be thrown at my ex-wife's house.

Strange Experience Still Brings Confusion

This story is a bit hard for me to discuss, but I believe it needs to be told. One night I woke up to darkness, looked at the wall and saw nothing, then looked at the digital clock and saw it read 3:30 a.m. This made sense, as I often woke up around this time to use the bathroom. Finally, I glanced at the window and turned to my side to go back to sleep, but it was then that I noticed something standing at the foot of my bed. Confused, I closed my eyes for a second. But when I opened them the figure was still there at the foot of my bed. My breathing became fast, in and out, gasping for air. We looked into each other's eyes, and I started to scream loud enough for my parents to hear, but they never came. The strange thing was that as soon as I stopped screaming a few seconds later, the shape went through my bedroom door, which was closed.

I am not sure what happened after that, but when I next opened my eyes, I could feel sunlight on my face. I got up and went downstairs, holding onto the handrail like always. We have a picture of the Virgin Mary in the kitchen, and when I sat down at the table, I noticed that what I had seen that night was the same shape as in the picture. Still shaken by my experience, I opened my laptop and looked for pictures of the Virgin Mary. The shape and the face were unmistakably what I had seen. At first, I thought it had been a dream, but I realized that this was the time I woke up every night; it could not have been a dream. My heart began to pound against my chest. I knew what I had seen. It took me a while to gather the courage to mention this experience to my parents. I had read stories of how the Virgin Mary appeared to people, but they were only stories, and I had been skeptical. After that night, my skepticism was gone.

Facial Nerve Surgery

I was doing quite a bit of reading about nerves and how they could be healed, and in one article I learned of a procedure where a muscle was removed from your inner thigh and transplanted into your face. I asked Dr. Oczkowski about this procedure, and he booked me an appointment with Dr. Bain, who specializes in that area.

I met Dr. Bain in his office at McMaster Hospital, and after we discussed my facial paralysis, he agreed to perform the surgery. The procedure had the potential to restore 90% of the original nerve function to the right side of my face, including movement.

The day of the surgery, I arrived at Hamilton General Hospital and checked in. I was told to change into a blue gown and lie on the bed that was there. I must say it felt awkward being naked except for this gown. A nurse came 10 minutes later and inserted an IV into my right arm, then after another five minutes a gentleman came and told my parents and I that he would take me to surgery. He verified my information and noticed the black lines on my face that the doctor had drawn earlier as I waited in bed. He explained that those lines were just for reference and that the marked side of my face would not be operated on. Then, leaving my parents behind, I entered the operating room. I was transferred onto the operating table, feeling my body hairs standing up in the cold room. I took note of the small group of people that would assist Dr. Bain with the surgery, then closed my eyes.

When I awoke, I was in a recovery room and my parents were standing at the foot of the bed. Dr. Bain then entered the room, walked up to me, and explained that the surgery had been a success. He had been able to do the bone realignment that should help my speech, and he would check up on me in a couple days to see how I was healing.

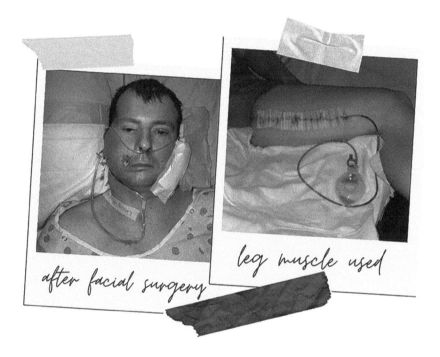

after facial surgery

leg muscle used

I was under too much medication to remember much of this time, especially the first day. I do remember having trouble sleeping on that first night and asking the nurse for a sleeping pill. She gave me one, but I could feel my head resisting and fighting the medication. I tried to close my eyes and could not, so I called the nurse and asked for some pain medication. I could see from the clock on the wall that it was 4 a.m. when she gave it to me, and I turned my head to the left and saw that my roommate who had been there earlier was gone. I started to freak out; I thought aliens must have taken him, and I cowered in the darkness. The only light I could see was in the hallway, and I had the urge to get up and run away, but I stayed in bed, fearing I wouldn't know what to do when I got out of the room. Then a stranger started chasing me. I started to scream, and a nurse showed up and asked what was wrong. I asked where my roommate had gone and why it had gotten darker; she explained that it was so I could sleep easier, and this calmed me down.

I was somber for a while, but I soon became frightened again. I thought the aliens were experimenting and this nurse was not really a nurse, just disguised as one. Again, I started to freak out and yell. The nurse rushed back into the room and asked what was wrong; I exploded with fear and panic. I told her I wanted to call my parents, and she explained that it was early in the morning and they were sleeping. But I insisted, crying, that I needed to call my parents.

She agreed and went to get a cell phone so I could call them. I was still crying when they answered the phone, but the conversation reassured me, and I was able to finally sleep soundly.

Over the next few days, I recorded myself talking and noticed that the bone realignment had improved my speech just like Dr. Bain said it would. I was extremely impressed and wondered why no one else had thought to try this relatively easy and safe procedure. It has been a couple months, and my bottom right facial nerve has started to function, although I am still waiting for the top right facial nerve to function again. A long scar on my inner left thigh marks where the muscle was taken, but I never experienced pain at the incision.

CHAPTER 20

An Injury and a Surprise

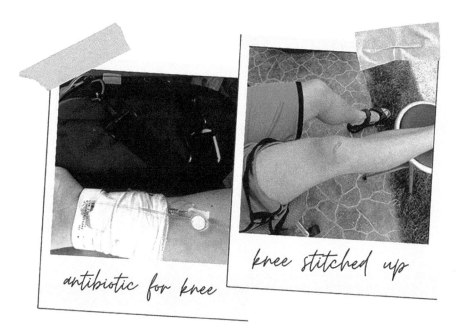

antibiotic for knee

knee stitched up

One day, I was going through my normal exercise routine on the hand-rail. I remember it was an especially warm day, and I felt the hot sun on my face. I wiped the sweat off my forehead and kept going, smiling away because everything was going well. But then I tried to take a step and my left leg was wobbly for some reason. Ignoring it, I brought my right foot toward my left foot, but it also became wobbly. I looked down and saw my legs were shaking. Then, without warning, my right leg gave out. I tried to grab the handrail, but I was too late. Everything seemed to go in slow motion as I bent my right knee to soften the fall; missing the wood I was standing on, I landed with my full body weight on a bent piece of metal that formed the walkway I was standing on. Surprisingly, no blood began to flow. *It's just a simple cut.* I called for my parents to help me up and showed them the cut. I thought it was no big deal, but when we investigated the wound, we saw that it went deep. My parents said a hospital visit would be in order. I refused to go, reminding them there was no blood, but in the end, they convinced to go to the hospital a few minutes' drive from their house. When we got to the emergency room, there was only one other patient waiting, and it was only a few minutes before my mom, and I were called in to see the doctor. After a quick observation, he concluded that stitches would be required to close the wound. He reached for a syringe and pointed it at the skin next to my wound. I closed my eyes and felt the poke of the cold needle penetrating my skin and the liquid dispersing underneath. The doctor pulled out the needle, and I felt a warmth spread all over my body. I opened my eyes and looked at my mom while the doctor prepared the thread. Then he said he was going to begin, and I felt heat rising on my forehead from fear as the doctor started to sew my wound closed. I kept eye contact with my mom, refusing to look down but feeling each time the doctor tightened the thread. After five stitches, I was relieved to learn that the ordeal was over.

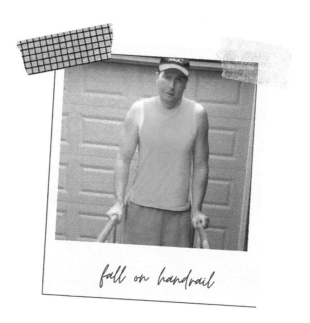

fall on handrail

Trike Surprise From My Neighbors

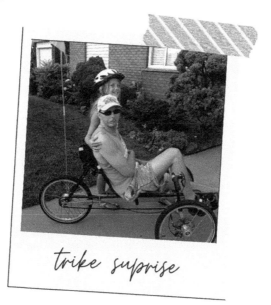

trike suprise

One day when we were sitting in the kitchen, my mom opened the door to go outside and noticed a trike—a bicycle with two wheels in front and one in the back—sitting in the yard. Apparently, our neighbors, Jim and Dawna Sawadski, had gotten me a super present that would let me travel the neighborhood without fear of falling. This was great; I could now go riding with my daughter to places like our local park.

I hopped onto the trike and began to ride down the street and around the neighborhood. It felt like the first time I had gotten a bike for Christmas as a kid; my world had just opened. The only difference was that this time there were no training wheels. I pedaled to extreme speeds, then stopped and felt the sweat gushing down my face; I was free, I could go places, I did not care.

My daughter and I biked to the park often, and I was able to watch as she played on the playground for the first time. We also biked around the neighborhood, looking at different houses; we even raced to see who would reach the house quicker. Unfortunately, I always lost, but this never bothered me. Thanks to my lovely neighbors and their gift, I could go places with my daughter, and that is all that mattered.

Shopping Cart From the Grocery Store

One day, my mom and I were talking about the walker and how our morning walks around the block were becoming easier. Our friend, Magda Skinner, arrived and joined in our conversation, saying why not just ask for a shopping cart? My mom and I pondered for a couple minutes and then decided to go to our local grocery store, Fortinos. We entered the store and asked for the manager, then asked him if I could have a shopping cart. We explained that it would greatly improve my ability to walk, and he agreed. Soon, the shopping cart was in the back of the SUV. We thanked the manager for his help and headed home.

Back at the house, I could not wait to try the shopping cart. It was ready for me on the driveway next to the car, and I went out to see it. I was brimming with excitement over the new chance to impress my mom. I gripped the cart and it felt stable; as I began to push it forward, I only felt a little unsteadiness. We reached the kitchen entrance door rather easily, and I sat on the bench outside to think about how I could improve the cart so that I could become more independent. My mom and Magda talked a little longer and she left, but we thanked her for her great idea.

My mom and I waited for my dad to get home from work to perfect the shopping cart. When he arrived, we showed it to him and explained what I thought would need to be adjusted. He removed the metal bar at the bottom so I would not hit my feet, and we placed different weight pieces in the cart to weigh it down, which would help me to control it better. Finally, it was done and ready for testing. My mom came out and we gave the cart its first walk around the block. I could feel all the neighbors watching as we strolled around the block with my improved shopping cart. It worked perfectly, and my mom and I started walking around the block every morning with the shopping cart. As I gradually improved, we subtracted weight to make it more difficult. Now, I do not use any weight in the cart—and I only use the heavy blue walker in the snow or on uneven terrain.

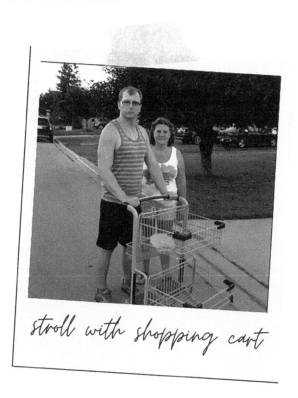

stroll with shopping cart

Moving to My Parents' New Place

As my indoor and outdoor movement and training expanded, my parents and I started discussing moving to a different place where I would have more space. After a while of searching, we finally found something outside the city; however, the house was small—even smaller than our current house. We decided to buy it and remodel it, and with some effort, it turned into a new house with easier and more comfortable wheelchair access and more space for me to move around. Now the only thing we were missing was the recreation center with the pool, but to remedy this, I purchased an outdoor pool so in the summer months I can train, and we all can relax.

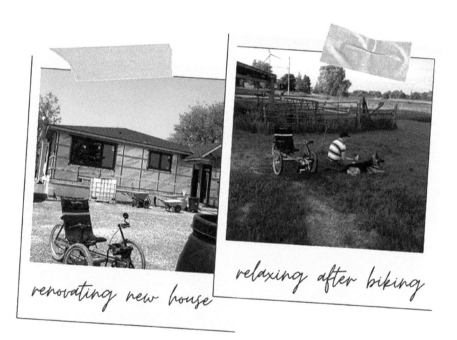

renovating new house

relaxing after biking

Surprising Nerve Pinch

My lower back started to hurt, but this seemed like nothing new; I was used to it hurting after I did certain exercises. So for a while, I pushed through the minor pain I felt. When the pain got worse, I stopped exercising altogether, thinking my muscles needed to recover, but the pain continued to worsen. I finally told my parents that my lower back was hurting, and they at first suggested the same thing I had been trying, but every hour the pain was increasing slightly. I decided to contact my neurologist, Dr. Oczkowski's, office to see if they had any suggestions. Only later would I learn that I had a pinched nerve; they simply emailed back that I should try over-the-counter pain medication. So I did just that; I swallowed the pills on a regular basis, and the more pain I felt in my lower back, the more pain medication I consumed. Soon I needed pain medication every night to close my eyes. This lasted for a couple of days, and my lower back pain continued to increase on an hourly basis. Sometimes even the medication could not completely mask the pain, and I would need to lie down, unable to do anything.

After a couple days, I remember waking up and needing assistance to go to the washroom. This really scared me; I remembered all too well what this was like and what came next. Of course, I could not lift myself from the toilet and had to call my mom to help me. I had a sharp twitch when I stood which caused my whole body to shake. I was very confused about what has happened, but I tried to ignore it. I wanted to resume my exercises, standing but not putting pressure of any kind on my lower back, so my mom helped me go downstairs to the handrail where I usually performed my standing exercises.

I stood there with both hands holding the bars of the handrail—left hand holding the left bar, right hand holding the right bar. I let go, and I could not believe my eyes: I could not hold any balance. I tried the walking exercise I was good at; well, let us just say I was swaying from side to side, bumping the bars constantly. With tears in my left eye and sadness in my voice, I called my mom. She came down and asked what was wrong, but I just said nothing, and she helped me get upstairs to sit on the couch. On the way up, I was overwhelmed with emotions about this experience. I cannot describe the devastated state I was in that day. I flopped down on the couch thinking about how this had set me back many years because I knew how long it had taken me to get to where I had been before this pain started, and now I had lost my progress. Despite everything I had been through, this felt like a new situation, and I honestly did not know how to approach it. I finally told my parents what I had lost, but their comforting words did not help; I knew deep down that this was a challenge I would have to face on my own.

But about an hour later, our lovely neighbor, Matt Bradbury, showed up at our doorstep. I told him what had happened to me, and he suggested a chiropractor and a massage. I was skeptical, but it was worth a try. As I sat in my wheelchair, he called a chiropractor not far from our house and booked an appointment for me to see him and get a massage right afterward.

The place was called Smithville Chiropractic Clinic, and the next day I showed up for the appointment. I was put onto the bed, and I explained my situation to the chiropractor; he then told me to lie down and he adjusted me with gentle cracking sounds in a variety of places. After 10 minutes of cracking, we were done. I had the massage right after the adjustment to relax my muscles, and after it was complete, we booked another appointment to continue.

I was on the couch at home later when I noticed that I felt different than usual. At first, I put it down to the unusually humid weather. But then I had to go to the washroom, and I noticed that my walking was different; I was able to hold better momentum on my own, not leaning so much on my mom. We reached the washroom and she left; later, I stood up without assistance. *Strange*, I thought. I sat back down, wanting to try this again. I stood up once more, again without needing to call for help. A gentle smirk came to my face; it seemed that this had helped, but I was skeptical. I told my mom I wanted to go downstairs to the handrail and see what I could do. First, I tried a simple exercise I could not do before, and to my surprise I did it on my first try. I then tried a more difficult exercise I was doing before this happened, and I was able to do it halfway. The smirk on my face grew wider; I was excited and surprised that this had helped so much after just one session and could not wait for the next session to see how far this could take me.

We arrived for my second appointment, and I excitedly told the chiropractor what had happened. By my estimate, I had already regained around 60% of the muscle function I had lost. He cracked me again for another three sessions before Christmas; in total, I regained around 80% of the movement I had lost. I remember thinking that this was not bad, just a small setback. After all, it had taken me two years to get to where I was, but with everything I now knew about physical therapy, I expected to be able to catch up much faster this time.

Finally Made it Happen

With the encouraging results from the chiropractor, I increased my training time dramatically. I noticed that some areas of my strength and balance were improving at different speeds. My balance was what took the longest to recover, but finally I wanted to try walking beside the handrail; I was already walking comfortably inside, but I had never attempted walking outside of it. I positioned myself at one end of the handrail on the right side of it, my feet on the ground, and my right-hand hovering over the bar just in case. I took a couple deep breaths, then I started with my right foot forward. I found I could hold the position. I moved my left foot just a little further than where my right foot was. I started to sweat, and I could feel my face getting red. But I could also feel the pressure to complete this, and I repeated the movement. Success—two steps down, 24 to go. I made my third step and noted with satisfaction that I was able to hold the movement I had made. I reached the halfway point and glanced back at how far I had walked, and I was already impressed with my accomplishment. I had the urge to continue what I had started to see how far I could go. I reached three-quarters of the way down the handrail, and my heart was crashing against my ribs. I started shaking and twitching from excitement; sweat began to form on my forehead and redness started to appear on my arms. Seeing that I was still holding on and so close to the end, I was panicking with excitement.

I've practiced more difficult exercises; I can do this, I said to myself. With tears in my eyes, I finally succeeded in walking the entire 26 small steps. I cannot explain the emotions I experienced upon completing this. After 11 years, I was finally able to walk without holding on. And not just one step, but 26. The hard part was accomplished, and the rest—getting back to normal walking—would just be icing on the cake.

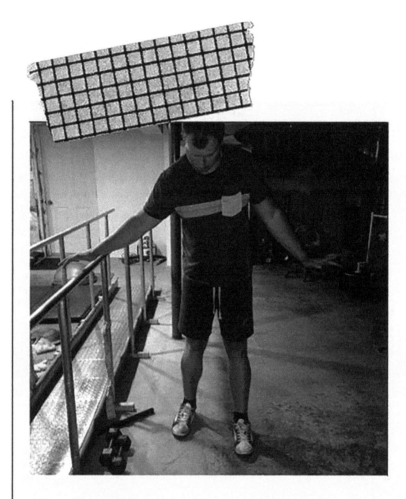

first time out June 2020

Isabella

My daughter was 17 months old when I was diagnosed. My time with her was ripped out of my hands, but thanks to the love and support of my friends and parents, I am reclaiming my life and my time with Isabella. Thank you especially to my parents; without them, I could never have gotten this far. And thank you to Isabella; she was always my reason for walking. That vision of us building a snowman, snow-flakes falling heavy on our faces and us opening our mouths to catch them, is what carried me through all those years. I know now that this will happen.

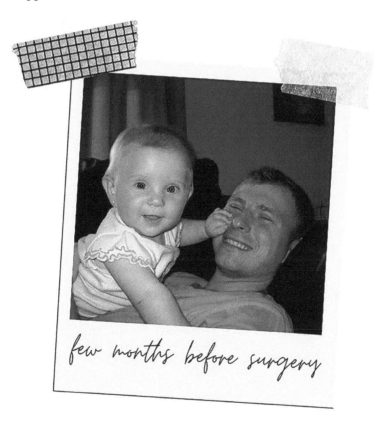

few months before surgery

TRAINING

I will be showing you exercises that worked for me. Will they work for you? Well worth a try! However, consult with your physician before starting, and please, if you experience any pain, stop the exercise immediately. Please be extra safe when doing standing exercises. Overall, be aware of your surroundings and always plan for the worst scenario.

With that said, as mentioned previously, I will be focusing on walking. There are a few areas we are going to be targeting, which, in my opinion, are the most used. They are as follows:

- Core
- Lower back
- Calves
- Quads
- Hips
- Abs
- Stabilizing muscles

By targeting these areas, we will also be targeting other muscles that help with each movement you perform. All areas play a role, but the ones listed are the essential ones. For best results, do exercises that require multiple muscles to perform a task.

I will try to explain the exercises that seem to be more effective for your balance recovery. I have adjusted the exercises for more improvement toward your body. You will learn and adjust the exercises for your needs. The point here is for you to notice how your body strength and balance work together. Once you grasp the concept, you will be doing exercises that you make up for your needs. Be patient with your improvement; it does take your body a long time to adjust to these movements that have not been performed for some time. Your body does heal, it just takes time. If you want your body to have extreme difficulty; just close your eyes.

CONTENTS

Rolling 132
    Laying on your back to roll 132
    Laying on your stomach to roll 132
Crawling on Your Knees 134
Your Quads 136
Knee Walking 138
Treadmill 140
Elliptical 141
Lower Back 142
Using Exercise Ball 144
BOSU® Wobble 145
Stationary Bike 146
Stability Muscles 147
Twists 149
Wheelchair 150
Hand Walkout 152
Abs 153
Extra Abs 155
Wall sit 156
Walking with Walker 157
Push-up 158
Lower Back, Core etc. 159
Support 160
Plank 161

Bridge 162
Core with Ball 163
Leg Pulls 164
Prepare for Standing 165
Standing 166
Standing Swing 167
Raising Hands 168
Little Squat 170
Ball Raise 171
Touch It 172
Angry Throw 173
Broom Sweep 174
Dress or Undress 175
Ball Bounce 176
Pick up 177
Wall Push Off 178
Exaggerate Bending 179
Water Drink 180
Bend Knee 181
Push Upwards 182
Hit or Touch 183
Touch 184
Shake 185
Step Tries 186
Place Your Leg 188
Feet Rock 190
Standing Movement 191
Rail Squat Pull 192
Leg Pull Up 193
Standing With Stick 194
Walking Kick 195
Pool Exercises 196
        Pool Standing 196
        Pool Abs 197
        Platform Walks 197

Noodle Walk.. 198
Dumbbell Hold 199
Reaching.. 200
True Walk 200

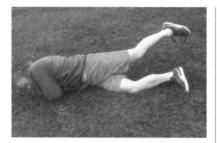

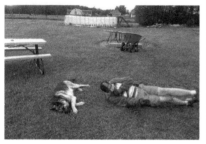

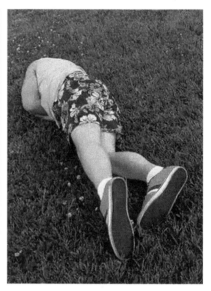

It was hard for me to roll at the beginning. This exercise can be done outside or indoors, wherever there is room. If there is not enough space, you may roll left and then right so you can complete one roll and then roll to the other side. You do control the way you roll with your legs, which in a way you are your steering wheel.

LAYING ON YOUR BACK TO ROLL

1. Lift the leg that is opposite from the way you want to roll, so if you want to roll to your left, lift your right leg.

2. With your right leg, cross your left leg, overreaching your left leg and down to the ground. At the same time, turn your torso to turn in that direction.

3. Use your leg weight to assist in turning, especially in the beginning until your muscles are strong enough and only momentum is used.

LAYING ON YOUR STOMACH TO ROLL

1. Lift the leg that is opposite from the way you want to

roll, so if you want to roll to your left, lift your right leg.

2. With your right leg, cross your left leg, overreaching your left leg and down to the ground. At the same time, turn your back to turn in that direction. Both positions are identical in movement. You are developing strength in the torso as well as learning how to use your body weight to your advantage. Do not be alarmed if this does not work right away and you just lift your leg but do not turn over. It took me a while before it began working; it is about learning the proper timing.

CRAWLING ON YOUR KNEES

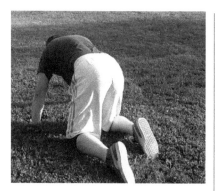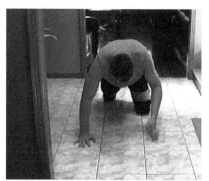

Crawling on my knees is one of my favorite exercises to do. This can be done everywhere, indoors or outdoors. It is an extremely basic exercise that is overlooked by most physiotherapists. You are going to develop the proper strength and balance through crawling before learning how to walk, just like a baby.

Get into position to crawl on your knees, hip width apart with your hands shoulder width apart, keeping your arms bent.

1. Go forward with your right hand first. Lift your right hand and place it forward half a foot. Once your right hand is on the ground, lift your left knee up and move it forward half a foot without your knee dragging.

2. Once the left knee is on the ground and forward the same distance as your right hand, move your left hand. Then lift your right knee once your left hand is on the ground and move your right knee forward the same distance as your left knee.

You may increase the difficulty by making bigger hand placements, more narrow or wider placements, or by adding weight on your back or ankle weights on your knees.

Once this becomes easy, start doing the reverse by crawling on your knees backward leading with your knee. Try to have your backside at 90°; however, this will take a while before your muscles are strong enough to hold that position while in motion. If you are confused, just ask someone to crawl on their knees and observe them. It is the same movement.

Eventually when you are strong enough, you will be crawling with your hands on the ground and your feet on the ground. The same rules apply as crawling on your knees.

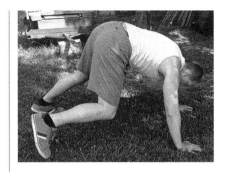

These muscles are mostly used when getting up from a seated position, like from a chair or a sofa. You need to strengthen these muscles to help you pull up. There is going to be more focus on this muscle, which needs to be strengthened before other supporting muscles assist. An example would be getting up from a sitting position to a standing position. You are using mostly your quads to lift your body up, then once your body is up, different muscles take over.

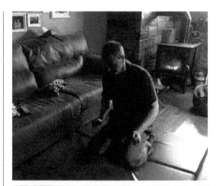

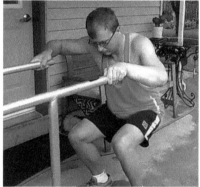

The most basic form of this exercise is to get on your knees, sit on the backs of your feet, then get back up to a 90° position.

If you want to combine this with a different form of exercise, simply try to hold your position at 90° once you lift yourself up from the backs of your feet. Do turning twists, catching a pillow in various positions, throwing the pillow back to different locations while maintaining your balance.

I recommend doing leg exercises with less repetition because they really cause muscle soreness and will affect your standing balance the next day.

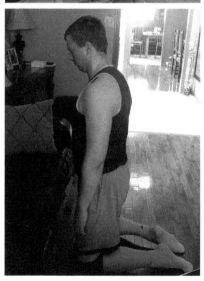

You can also just stretch your quads by going from a kneeling position and slowly moving to a sitting position.

KNEE WALKING

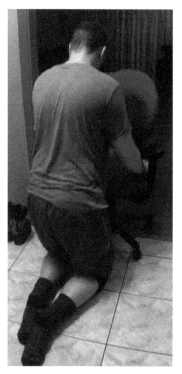

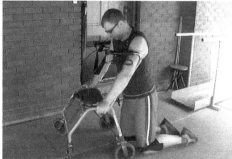

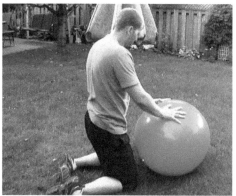

In the beginning, I would recommend using a chair that does not move.

1. Stand on your knees, close to the chair at 90°.
2. Lift the chair and set it back down half a foot forward, keeping your hands on the chair.

You are going to try to make a step with your knees. This will be difficult in the beginning.

1. Shift your weight on the opposite knee, feeling that the body weight is on that knee.
2. Once you feel the weight, lift your other knee slightly forward. You may drag in the beginning, but try to keep

your knee off of the floor and prevent it from dragging.

Use your hands that are on the chair for balance. You may lean a bit on the chair until your muscles get stronger (avoid leaning on the chair too much and stand at 90°).

Once this becomes easy, increase your difficulty depending on the items that you possess. The next step will be using something with wheels, for example, you may push a walker forward half a foot or lift the walker half a foot. Repeat what you did in the beginning. Once this has become easy, you may try an exercise ball which you can roll half a foot or pick up the exercise ball and place it half a foot in front of you.

The final step is to kneel 90° without anything for support. At first, try to make the steps ridiculously small and make them larger until this is easily accomplished. For extra fun, hold some weights in your hands to make it more difficult for your body to adjust, just like in real life.

I would suggest having a safety harness attached when you are using a treadmill.

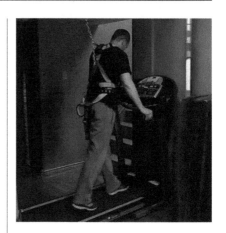

Begin with five minutes each day on the treadmill so your muscles get used to the new leg movement. You can eventually increase your time to 10 minutes then 20 minutes.

Now your legs are ready for some difficulty. First, start with the height three levels higher than flat, then after 10 minutes, lower it each time. You can also try moving your hands in different positions.

Once this is completed easily, you may increase the time or adjust the machine to make it more difficult. You can also confuse your legs and do flat, high, and middle settings for extra challenge. Remember, if it is too easy, you are not improving. This goes for every exercise.

ELLIPTICAL

The elliptical is a particularly good exercise to get your body, muscles, joints, and especially hips, moving. Start off with a short amount of time and slowly increase once it becomes too easy. Also, you may increase the difficulty of resistance. Please wear a safety harness just in case.

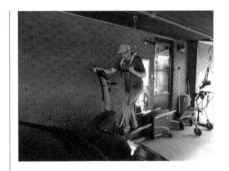

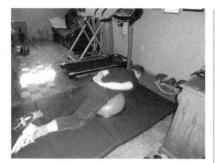

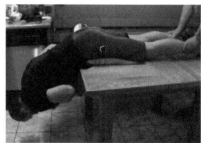

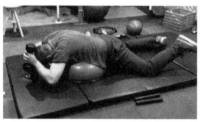

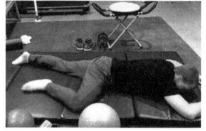

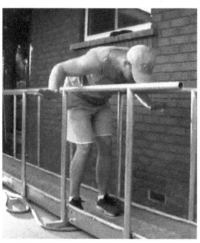

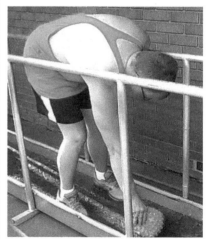

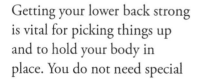

Getting your lower back strong is vital for picking things up and to hold your body in place. You do not need special machinery to develop this muscle to meet your needs.

The most basic exercise for the lower back is laying on your stomach with your arms on the side of your body while trying to lift your chest. If you want more difficulty, simply adjust your arm placement. You can even hold something in the air and do the exercise.

The next level up is to lay on the BOSU® ball and do the same as above.

Lastly, you may combine this exercise by picking something up off the ground or bending your chest up to 90°, or even lower, and then back up. You may have your knees bent or straighten your knees to increase the difficulty and have a stretch.

Adjust to your needs, but if standing, be with a partner or have something to grab on to just in case.

As with the last picture, lay on your stomach and bring your knee up, then return down. Finally, do the same with the opposite side, but make sure you are wearing slippery clothes.

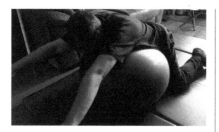

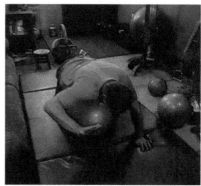

The exercise above also incorporates your stability muscles that prepare you when you are on an uneven surface and you need to pick something up. The point here is to have something unstable underneath on your stomach, and your body will need to adjust and adapt to your movement. With this exercise you are targeting multiple muscles.

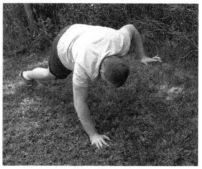

Lift your arms, place the exercise ball as shown above, then lift your chest. You may also use the ball to lean on when you lift your knee off the ground, using your hands for stability.

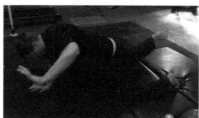

Eventually, you will be attempting this exercise without the ball as support.

BOSU® WOBBLE

Depending on your BOSU® ball, you want to turn it over with the flat side up. Get into a push-up position and place your forearms to the handles. From there, gently rock left and right until this position becomes easy. When it does, you will be more aggressive with rocking side to side. If you want to make it more difficult, just use narrow foot placement.

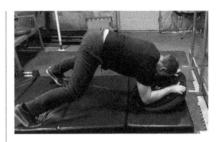

STATIONARY BIKE

This exercise gets taken for granted, but it works out multiple muscles that control your movement. For example, when you pedal you are constantly shifting your weight and your body must adjust for this movement.

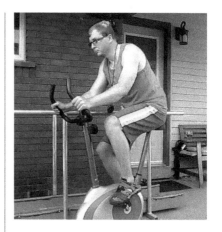

To make it more difficult, hold the handles in different places, hold with one arm, or don't hold anything, which will take some time.

Increase your time, resistance, or speed for more difficulty.

For your safety, I would place the stationary bike close to a wall where you can lean or rest if needed.

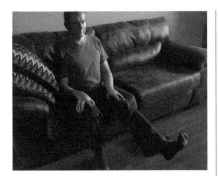

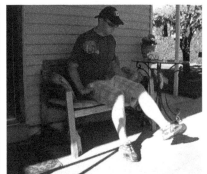

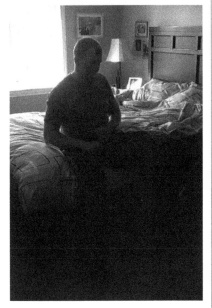

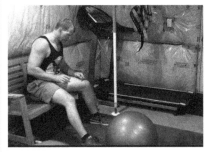

1. In the beginning, I would suggest sitting on a soft mattress with your feet touching the ground. Then, while making slight movements to get your body off-balance, your muscles will work harder to keep you from falling.

2. Once the mattress becomes easy, move to something more difficult—like an air mattress

The point here is to sit on something unsteady. By doing so, you engage your stability muscles which help you keep your balance. These muscles are the ones we want to get stronger.

slightly depleted of air—to make it more unsteady.

3. If once again this becomes easy, sit on a balance disk, and create movement. You can kick a rolling ball or just lift one leg up while keeping balanced. You may turn side-to-side or clap your hands or you can pick something up from the ground to make it more challenging.

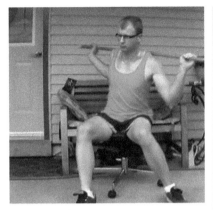

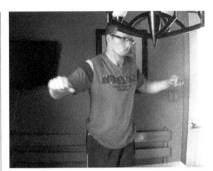

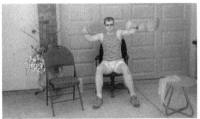

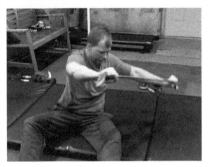

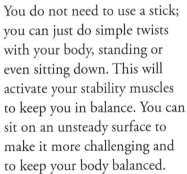

You do not need to use a stick; you can just do simple twists with your body, standing or even sitting down. This will activate your stability muscles to keep you in balance. You can sit on an unsteady surface to make it more challenging and to keep your body balanced.

You may do twisting standing up; you can use the ball or just twist. If standing, just be safe. It is best to stand near a wall so you can lean on it in case you lose your balance.

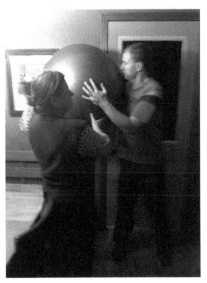

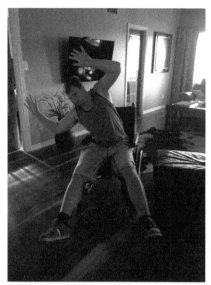
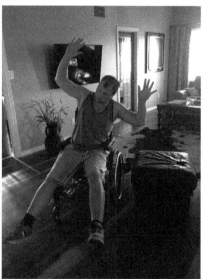
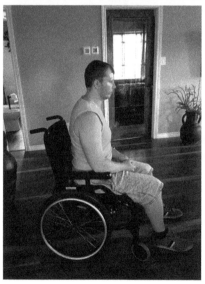
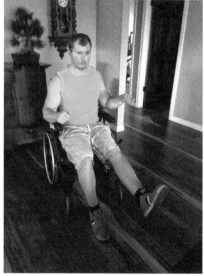

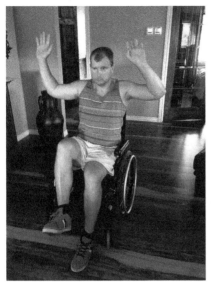 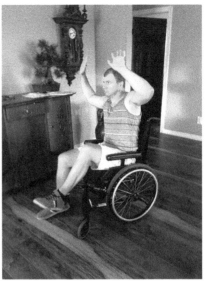

Sitting in your wheelchair or just a chair can provide you a workout.

1. By simply not leaning on your chair, you are developing your back muscles that stabilize your back.
2. Attach a weight to your ankle to increase the difficulty. Lift your leg and switch legs if you want more of a challenge. You can also perform twist movements and circular movements with your torso. You can also do this exercise sitting on a soft surface like a mattress with your hands up.

HAND WALKOUT

There are multiple variations of this exercise, but basically, keep your feet grounded and crawl with your hands going forward above your head, then back down. If this is too difficult at first, you can start this exercise by kneeling and then arching to form an upside down 'U'.

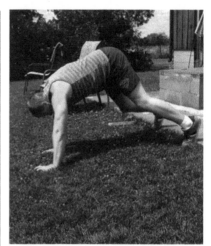

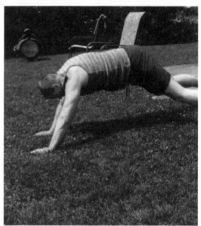

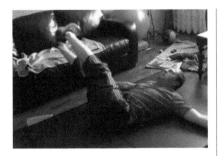 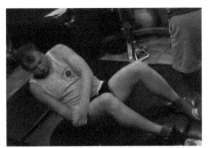

I did not do a lot of ab exercises since they are all indirectly activated while performing different workouts that target your midsection.

The above exercise is simple to do.

1. Lay on your back.
2. Place your hands on your side for balance.
3. Lift your legs together up to 90° and move them slowly side-to-side.

If you need extra support for your feet, have someone hold them down so they do not slide. The wider apart your feet are, the easier it is.

1. Have your knees bent with the hands together and move them with your torso side-to-side.
2. You may have variations here by adding more resistance like holding weights in your hands.

To do these simple leg lifts, lay on your back and lift your legs up as high as possible. Of course, there are variations like having your legs together or apart for different levels of difficulty. You can also hold a medicine ball between your legs with the weight.

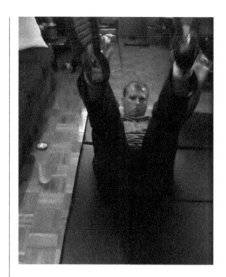

To prevent arching your back, keep your head up and do not drop your legs all the way down. When your back begins to arch, do not continue to lower your legs as this will cause lower back injury.

EXTRA ABS

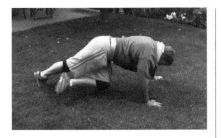 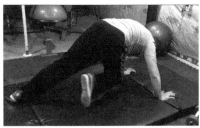

Get into a plank position with your hands on the ground. Make sure to keep your elbows bent a little. This exercise works different sets of muscles, including your abs.

In this position, place one leg underneath you and across to the other side. Another variation is bringing your knee towards your chest and back out.

WALL SIT

Position yourself against the wall in a sitting position and have your knees at 90°. You can adjust the angle for different resistance as well as your feet placement.

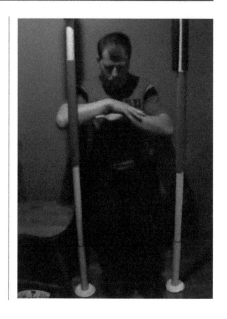

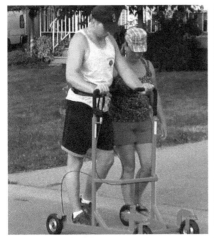
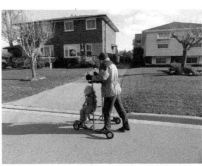
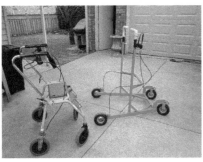
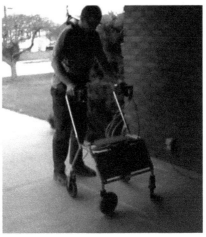

If you really want to target the muscles and recover muscle memory, practicing walking is very essential.

1. Start walking using a platform walker and have someone with you just in case.
2. To increase the difficulty, add ankle weights. If you are comfortable, walk by yourself around the block, going further each time.
3. If the platform walker is no longer challenging, move into a normal walker which is weighed down for more control.
4. Remove the weights from the walker and practice with someone there just in case.

This is an exercise that helps develop strength in different muscle groups, preparing you for other exercises.

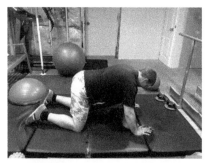

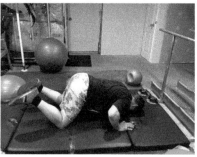

1. The easier version of a push up is to go on your knees, then down to the ground with your chest.
2. When close to the ground, push back up into the starting position.

Placing your hands or knees closer together makes it more difficult. If this is too easy, you can do a normal push up by straightening your legs and balancing on your toes instead of your knees.

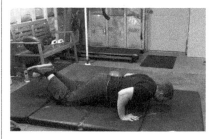

The more aggressive variation is to go down extremely close to the ground and then forward as much as possible. Do this on your knees or in normal push-up position. This will indirectly target your core while challenging your upper body strength.

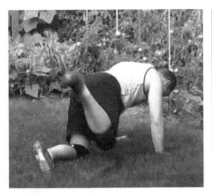 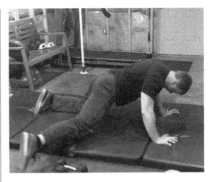

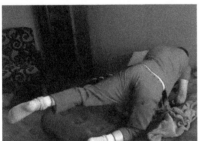 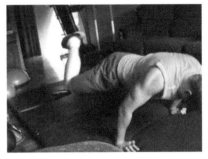

While in the crawling position, the easier version is to lift your leg up behind you. This will target multiple muscles especially your core, lower back, and legs. Make sure to flex your abdomen. Another variation is to move your legs to the side instead of behind you. If you make the bottom surface unsteady it will make your stability muscles work their hardest.

Challenge your core and arm strength by removing one of your hands that is supporting you. You can be on an uneven surface for an extra challenge which will also activate your smaller stabilizing muscles that prevent you from falling.

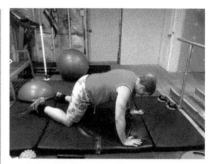

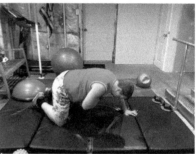

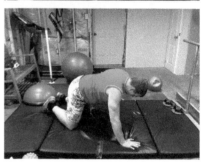

PLANK

There are a couple of variations
of this exercise, but I just
did the following. No need
to complicate things.

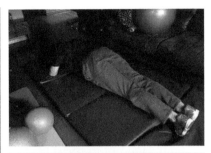

1. Get into the push-up position
   with your legs straight on
   your toes and your hands
   straight or on your forearms.
2. Hold this position while
   flexing your abs and keeping
   yourself in somewhat
   of a straight line.
3. Rock with your feet forward
   and back. You can have your
   legs in different locations.

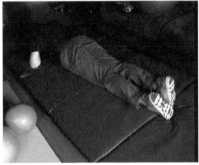

This is quite a simple exercise that you can do pretty much anywhere. There are multiple variations of this workout which you can adjust to your needs.

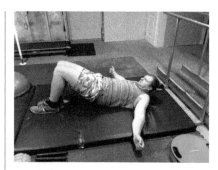

1. Lay on your back and place your arms out to the side.
2. Place your feet on the ground and lift your lower back up. The closer your feet are to your body, the easier it is.

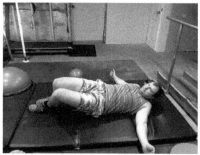

3. Hold your position for a few seconds, then go back down.
4. To increase difficulty, move your legs side-to-side slowly. If your feet are touching together the exercise is more difficult.
5. You can go even further by resting one leg on the ground and having the other in the air moving side-to-side.

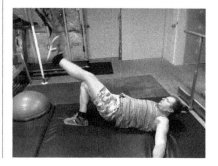

CORE WITH BALL

1. Hold a medicine ball weighted-in between your knees and go side-to-side.
2. If you really want to challenge your core with the stability muscles, do a bridge with your legs on the exercise ball. With both legs, go side-to-side with your legs on the ball, then do one leg at a time.
3. If you feel comfortable, move your arms that are supporting your body and place them at your side.

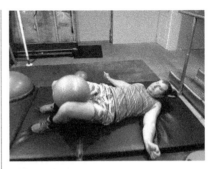

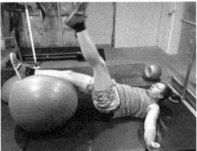

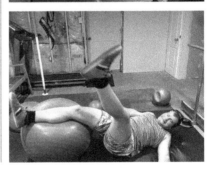

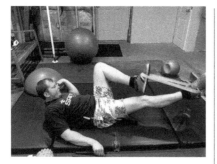 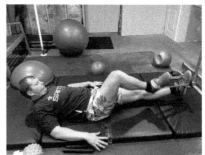

The effectiveness of this exercise is underestimated. Leg pulls activate the muscles required for pulling something.

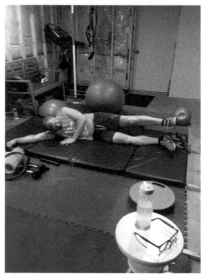

1. Lay on your back and place a resistance band mid-way on your feet.
2. Push one leg out and keep the other leg bent to resist the pulling of the band from the other leg.
3. Switch legs.

Depending on the stretchiness of the resistance band, it will be either harder or easier to pull.

These are some ideas about doing some leg exercises.

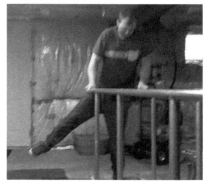

PREPARE FOR STANDING

I found this exercise highly effective in preparing for the standing position.

1. Place your hands on the chair handles. Holding down the handles helps you gain the balance needed to perform the motion to get up.
2. With your legs underneath the chair, raise up using your legs and hold until your arms are straight.
3. Try holding this position without holding on to the handles.
4. Go back down.

You may increase the difficulty with your feet placement. Either place them further out from the chair or in a narrower position.

If this exercise is quite easy for you, you may combine it with a different one. The higher your seating placement, the easier it is to get up. If you are practicing by yourself, have something to grab on to just in case you lose your balance.

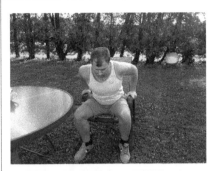

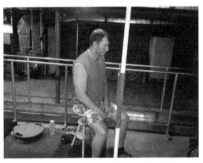

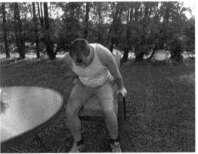

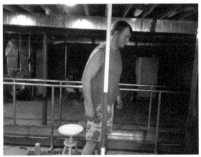

STANDING

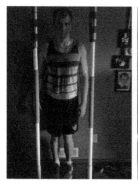 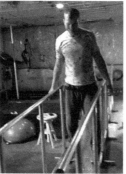 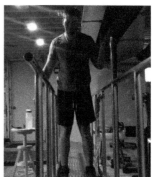

Depending on your level, I am assuming you are able to stand, but if not, you are still going to benefit as some of these exercises will help you in the future when you are able to stand. You are trying to develop the smaller muscles that hold your body together when making a small movement. The role of these smaller muscles is to prevent you from losing your balance.

Your muscles need to get used to your body weight and the movement that accompanies it.

Most exercises I perform are in my railway, which you may do without, but just be safe. I do not want you to get injured by losing your balance and falling. With each exercise be extremely cautious of your surroundings and if you fall, fall safely.

1. Stand in the railway, holding something sturdy with your hands, legs shoulder width apart.
2. Release your grip.
3. Slowly shift your weight onto the right leg, then left, feeling the weight of your body on that leg.
4. To make things more challenging, put your legs closer together as you go. You can also try putting one foot in front of the other and vice versa.

The point here is to get your muscles to learn the weight that is going to be applied.

Do not worry if the narrow foot placement is exceedingly difficult, you will get it in time.

STANDING SWING

1. While standing, slowly do
   gentle swings with your arms.

   You are teaching your brain
   how your small muscles are going
   to be reacting to this situation.

2. Do more aggressive swings.
3. Incorporate holding weights.
4. Do different standing
   positions with your feet.

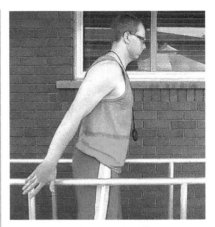

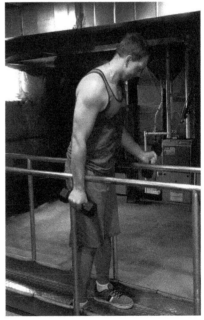

RAISING HANDS

You want your body to properly react when you are raising an object with your hands.

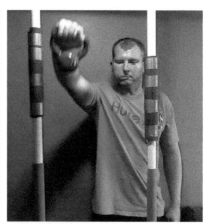

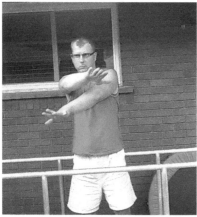

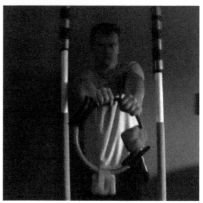

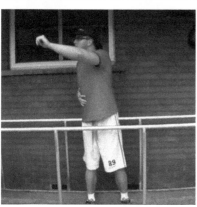

4. Lift your arms together to different locations.
5. Lift both arms above your head with both arms pointing in different directions.
6. Include weights when you lift your arms.

1. While standing, lift one arm in the air.
2. Switch arms.
3. Lift your arms together up above your head.

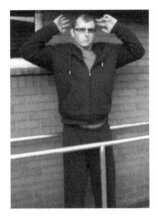 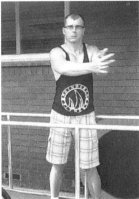 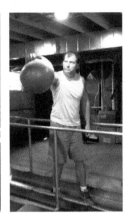

You want to get your muscles learning how to keep you balanced when you have different placements of your arms and different feet positions when you are standing. The images above give you some ideas of the different things that can be applied.

LITTLE SQUAT

1. While standing, bend your knees a little bit.
2. Go back up to standing.
3. Use different foot placements.
   Depending on how you do your squat you can have your arms forward holding a weight or holding a medicine ball, which can also train your lower back muscles.

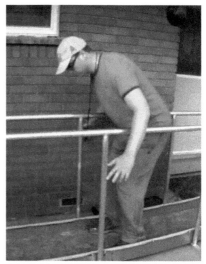

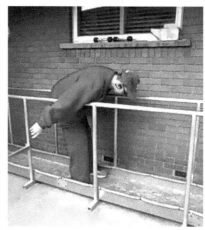

BALL RAISE

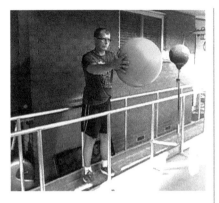

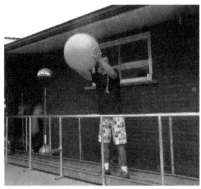

This does not have to be a ball; you can use something soft that has a bit of weight to it.

While holding the ball and standing, lift the ball in different directions.

If you have a partner, they can hand you the ball at different locations, then you can grab the ball from them and give it back. When you feel comfortable, your partner throws the ball and you try to catch it. Pointing to different locations also challenges your body and activates smaller muscles.

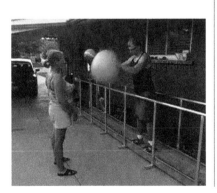

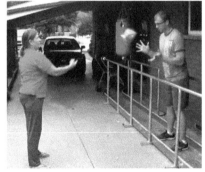

TOUCH IT

Hit something with force or just pretend to hit something in the air and it will cause the smaller muscles to stabilize your movement. It is a good idea to touch something that is moving because not only do you practice your balance, but you are also developing a better coordination by touching a moving object.

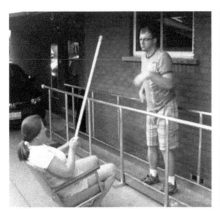 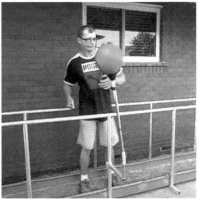

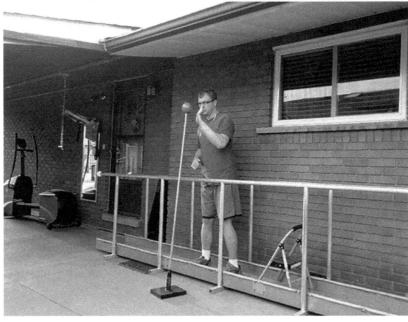

ANGRY THROW

This exercise will get your whole body shaking and force your stability muscles to be immediately activated.

1. Hold a medicine ball or a pillow.
2. Raise up with your hands, holding the medicine ball or pillow above your head.
3. With a forceful motion, throw the pillow or your medicine ball to the ground.
4. Pick it back up.

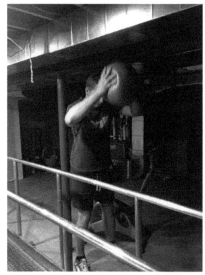

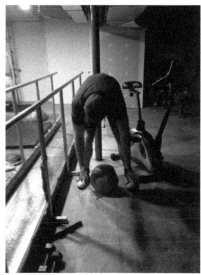

BROOM SWEEP

This is a unique exercise that involves a broom and sweeping. Sweep some dirt into a pile or just pretend you are sweeping. For extra difficulty, attach a weight or hold the broom straight with your arm and point to different locations.

1. Grab a broom.
2. Stand.
3. Sweep away.
4. Switch hands.

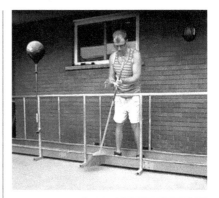

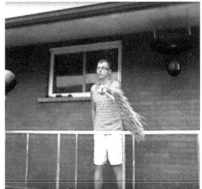

DRESS OR UNDRESS

This is a challenging
exercise involving getting
dressed or undressed.

1. Stand up.
2. Put your sweater on or off.
3. Or, you can unzip and remove
   it and put it back on.

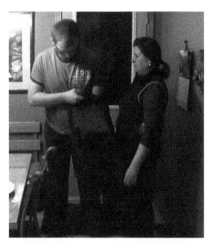

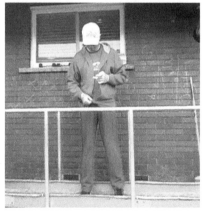

BALL BOUNCE

1. Bounce or hit a ball, or just pretend you are if no partner is available.
2. While standing, bounce or hit the ball back to the person. If you don't have a partner, just pretend.

This exercise is involving your stability, which will prepare you for the walking movement. Your focus is to develop these muscles to hold your movement.

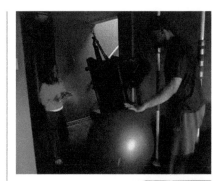

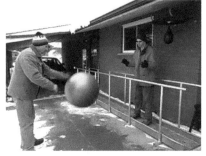

PICK UP

Depending on your ability, pick something up from the standing position.

1. While standing, bend down and grab the item from the floor.
2. Bring it up to you.
3. Place it back down.
4. Make it heavier if possible.
5. Use one hand for more difficulty.

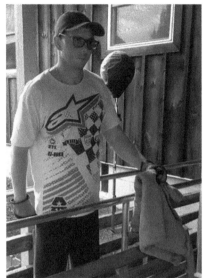

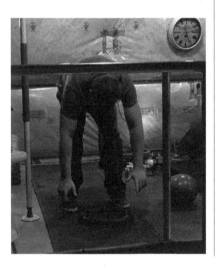

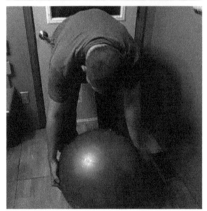

WALL PUSH OFF

Lean against the wall with just your shoulder blades so that you avoid pushing off from your hips. While leaning against the wall you are going to go into your standing position by thrusting forward. Please do this exercise in a narrow hallway and have someone there or have something to grab just in case. For more challenge, lean further away from the wall.

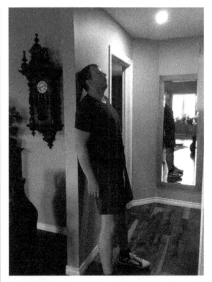

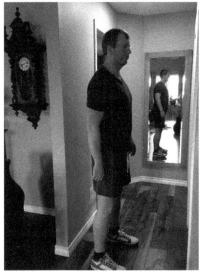

EXAGGERATE BENDING

This is a good balance exercise for your body to hold you together if you have a situation where you get an unusual stance.

1. While standing, bend far to one side.
2. Repeat for the other side.
3. When you are feeling comfortable, include holding something in your hands.
4. When you are bending forward, lean side-to-side with your body.

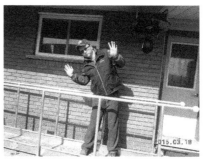

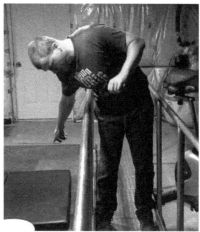

This is an incredibly good exercise to test the improvement in your balance. Basically, let someone pass you a glass of water and raise it up to your face and try to drink from it. Try not to spill anything.

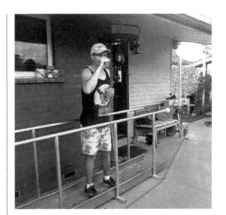

1. While standing, take a glass of water.
2. Try to drink from it without spilling.
3. Give it back or place it down.

BEND KNEE

With this exercise you want to bend your knee with one leg, shifting your weight onto the other leg. When you have a bent knee, you are going to point on your toes on the ground with that leg.

1. While standing, bend the knee that is going to be used.
2. Shift your weight to the other leg.
3. Point your toes with your leg that is bent.

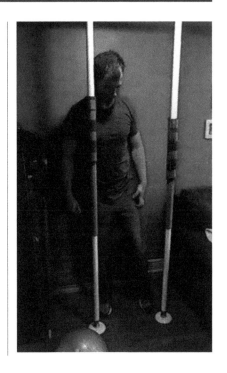

PUSH UPWARDS

1. Get into a plank position onto your forearms.
2. Raise up with your arms.
3. Hold the position.

You can adjust your arm placement for more difficulty. This tests your strength, your balance, and it activates smaller muscles.

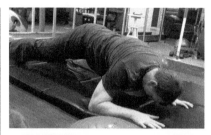

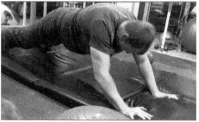

HIT OR TOUCH

Not only are you challenging your balance when standing, but you are also practicing your coordination in aiming where you want to punch or touch the object.

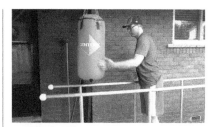

1. While standing, hit or touch a moving object if you have one.
2. If possible, use full punching or touching force against the object.

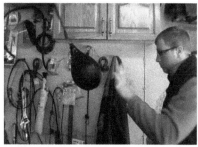

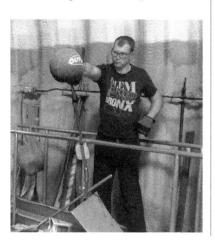

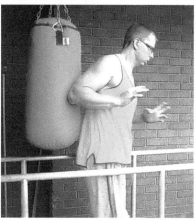

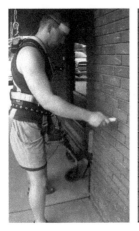 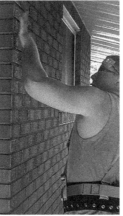 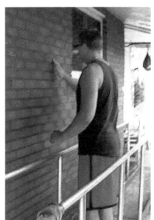

Focus on the item you want to touch. Touch Wall going up, then down, and then switch hands. For an even better workout, draw something with chalk. If not, have points on the wall and touch them one by one going upward.

1. While standing, touch a point on the wall and return.
2. Touch about five points, going higher each time.
3. Repeat with both hands at the same time.

SHAKE

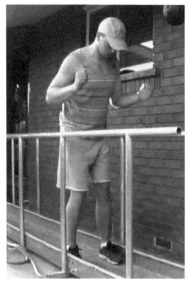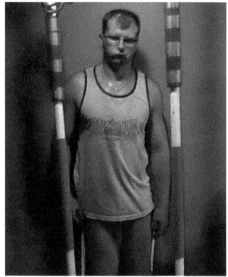

Stand with different foot placements and simply make your body shake. Be very unsteady here, which in turn activates your stability muscles that try to keep you in balance. In doing so, you are making these muscles stronger.

While standing, keep your feet shoulder width apart and shake by bending your knees a bit and raising your arms. Shake your head and different body parts.

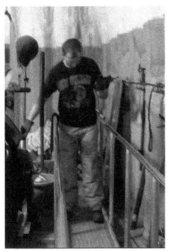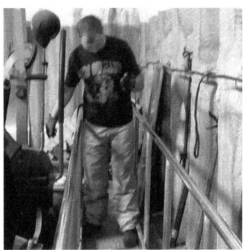

When you feel your body weight on your supporting leg, lift your opposite leg forward. After this is accomplished, you may do twists or slight movements to get you off balance. You want to activate your stability muscles to keep you in balance. You can also practice this with your foot a little upfront and return movement to the starting position and switch legs. For the best control, lead with your knee and not your foot. Remember, you are in control of where your foot lands. This exercise will take a lot of trial and error to find what is best for you.

This is very similar to walking on your knees which you have hopefully been practicing. With this exercise and walking on your knees, you are able to cheat a little by leaning forward. But with walking in a walker, treadmill, or in a swimming pool, you are not able to cheat—or at least I have not been able to.

If you look closely at people walking, you will see that when they take a step their shoulder goes down a little as well. That is when a shift of weight has occurred. The torso is used without their knowledge for this. Right now, you must do it manually, and sometimes you cheat by leaning one way using the body weight to your advantage. I personally do not like to walk like a duck and try to minimize the leaning if possible. Once your muscles can hold your movement, your leaning will disappear without you even thinking, the movement will just happen.

It takes loads of training. Since you have not used these muscles in a long time, the only way to really target what is needed is to make the movement with no machinery assistance (unless necessary) for short-term; you must do this move yourself to develop the muscle strength needed. That is why if possible, I recommend using a walker constantly to strengthen not just the legs but a whole bunch of muscles that assist with walking.

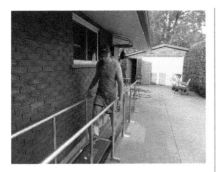

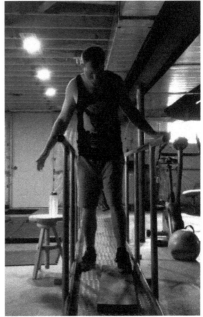

Same as the exercise above, you are going to be shifting your body weight onto your supporting leg. You may cheat a little by leaning slightly forward which helps you with the weight shift. Once you feel the weight on your left leg, lift and place the right leg higher and hold it there and vice versa. Of course, if you want to increase the difficulty, you can place your leg higher or start with a narrower foot position. When the foot lands in this position, you can do twists, shaking things to get you off balance. In return, you are practicing keeping your balance from a violent movement that is occurring. Do not worry if your foot placement is off; you want to practice multiple positions.

1. While standing, keep your legs shoulder width apart.
2. Shift your body weight onto the leg that is going to stay still.
3. Raise your other leg forward and place it on something higher.
4. Hold the position.
5. Try to go off balance, but fight to keep standing.

Standing Movement

1. While standing, move your hands up and return.
2. Move a single hand up and return.
3. With straight arms, clap and return.
4. Attach weights to your arms to make it harder.

FEET ROCK

When you stand, you stand on your toes and your heels. Practicing small movements with your feet is important in learning how to walk.

1. While standing, keep your legs shoulder width apart.
2. Go on to your heels, then your toes.
3. You can also place your feet in different positions or just tap with your feet.

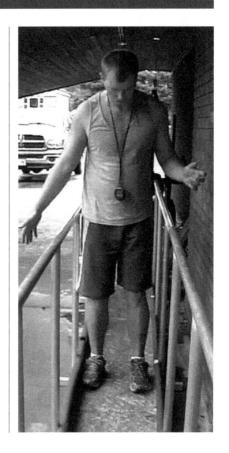

STANDING MOVEMENT

1. While standing, move your hands up and return.
2. Move a single hand up and return.
3. With straight arms, clap and return.
4. Attach weights to your arms to make it harder.

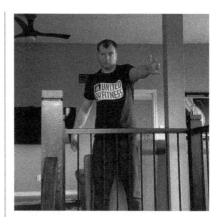

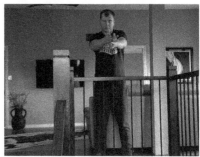

RAIL SQUAT PULL

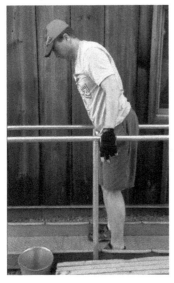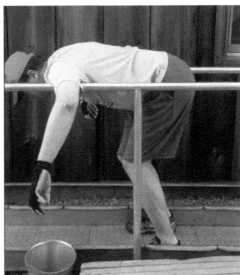

For a rail squat pull, you will need a railway like in the picture. The point of this exercise is to use your core and stability muscles to squat down, then push out and reverse.

1. When doing the squat, make sure you go straight down to your armpits.
2. Using your core, slide forward using the bars for support.
3. To complete the task, slide back in and stand up.

LEG PULL UP

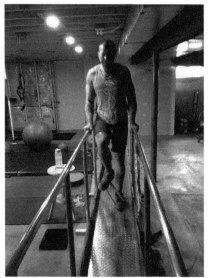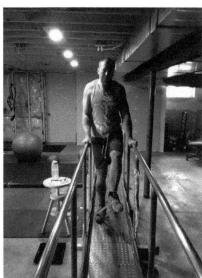

1. While standing, hold on to two things with your hands for support.
2. Put an elastic band or weights on your feet.
3. Lift your leg up with your knee straight.
4. Go back down and switch legs.

For this exercise, I find that rubber bands work better because not only do you have to lift your leg up, but you also have to fight to keep it up and stable.

STANDING WITH STICK

Just like raising your arms, you may do the same thing with an object that makes it more difficult for you to keep balance. I have used a stick, but you may use something else. While standing with the stick, you can try different variations of movement like holding it up with two hands, moving it side-to-side with one hand, or even adding some weights to it.

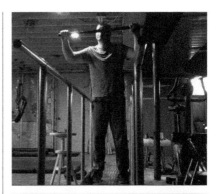

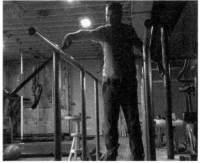

WALKING KICK

If you are at this stage, try making small steps in the beginning and bigger ones as you go.

As you learned earlier, the same task is applied, but this time when moving your leg forward, you are going to be kicking an object. I was gently kicking a board, but you may kick an air depleted ball or a pillow. You do not want something to go far as your steps are exceedingly small.

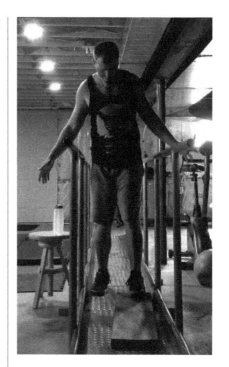

1. While standing, keep your feet are shoulder width apart.
2. Shift your body weight onto your still leg.
3. Move the other leg forward, kicking the object in the same motion.

POOL EXERCISES

I have found that doing physiotherapy in the swimming pool is amazingly effective. You can do most exercises that require standing in the swimming pool. You have additional resistance when you are standing or walking that is not felt by people without a balance issue. You can use the water for support using different floating objects or just your hands. It also eliminates some of your body weight depending on the water depth.

If you have access to a swimming pool through a recreation center or at home, I suggest you take advantage of it and feel the difference for yourself. When you are in the water, if you lose your balance, your falling speed is reduced with your weight. You are much easier to catch compared to when not in water.

If necessary, wear a life jacket until you are fully comfortable.

POOL STANDING

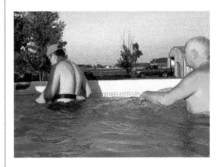

Like I said earlier, you can do pretty much all the exercises that required you to stand. Same rule applies, you want your stabilizing muscles to keep you balanced while you are trying to go off balance. I am not going to be listing the same exercises as above, just some things to give you an idea. You are your own doctor and you know what needs to be worked and how to make improvements along the way.

For best results, be in warm water since it relaxes your muscles. Do not overdo it the first time; increase your repetitions each day like any workout you do.

Stand in a corner of the pool. Feel the water moving and trying to get you off balance, your stabilizing muscles will be activated for you to stand.

Some examples of things you can do are:

1. Gentle squats or aggressive squats.
2. Different foot placements.
3. Step position with one foot in front and the other foot behind.
4. Use your hands to create resistance by pushing the water in and out underwater with your hands.
5. Let the other person create waves to increase your holding balance difficulty.

Remember, you can use your hands to support yourself with pushing the water in and out of the water.

POOL ABS

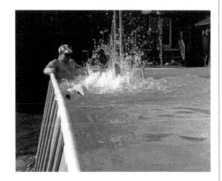

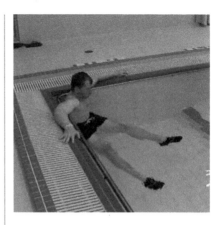

Get in the corner of the pool and place your arms on each side for support. You can do bicycle movements forward and backward and you can bring in your knees to your chest and back out. There are multiple variations of swimming pool ab exercises which you are not able to do outside of the swimming pool including:

PLATFORM WALKS

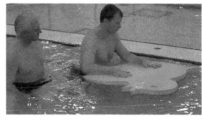

In the beginning, use something quite big to support your body. Avoid leaning on it so it does not go underwater. If you are putting too much pressure on it you will notice the water going onto your supporting item and it will go under causing you to lose your balance.

When I was noticeably confident in my ability that the platform was not going to sink, I placed a cup filled with water in the middle of the platform. This would show me physically if I was using too much support, and if so, the cup would fall.

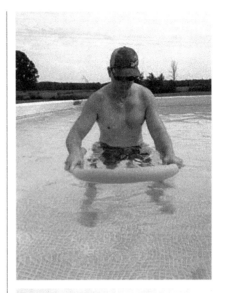

1. Stand at the edge of the pool by the wall.
2. Start to slowly make small steps with the platform in front of you.
3. Once confident, make larger steps and move faster.
4. Try walking with a smaller platform, making sure it doesn't sink.

NOODLE WALK

It is a good idea to confuse your body while in the water. Keep challenging your balance to improve.

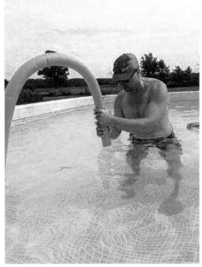

This exercise is just like the platform walk but with a noodle instead for support. Hold the noodle in different hand position to increase the challenge.

DUMBBELL HOLD

I personally like foam dumbbells since they not only provide support, but you can have a workout simply by submerging the dumbbell underwater.

1. Walk with two dumbbells above the water.
2. Move the dumbbells in different positions, for example, wider or narrower.
3. Try using one dumbbell in one hand, then switching.
4. Once you get more comfortable, increase the speed.

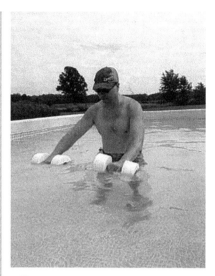

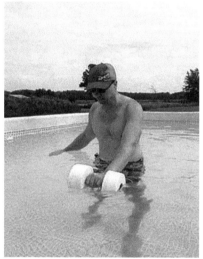

REACHING

You may reach for floating objects or touching something causing a twist.

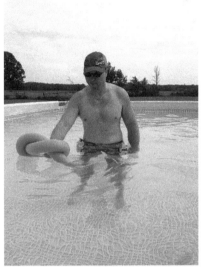

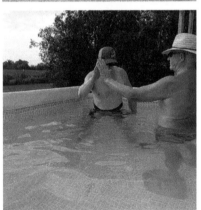

TRUE WALK

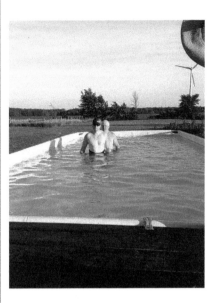

It is time to test your walking. You will notice that walking has a bit of difference from the outside of the swimming pool. There is support from the water plus the reduction in your body weight from the water. In the beginning, just make small steps until you feel comfortable to make larger ones. You cannot really notice the shift in body weight, you just make the movement automatically.

Your hips will take over
without you thinking about
this movement that you want
to accomplish when you are
out of the swimming pool. It
is extremely hard to explain
this, but you will notice
the difference when you are
in the swimming pool.

To make it easier for my
parents, I had a black belt
around my waist, which they
could grab onto and catch
me if I lost my balance.

1. Start at the end of the
   pool by the wall and
   start slowly moving.
2. Attempt making small steps.
3. Increase the size of steps.
4. Increase the speed.

FAQ

I wanted to answer some questions that you may have regarding my story and the physical therapy after reading the book.

Q: Will I recover?
A: This is extremely hard to answer; you will certainly improve. No one can answer this question because there are too many variables that may complicate the recovery, but from my personal experience, I will say yes. When people said, "No, you cannot," I practiced until I could.

Q: Why don't you mention your family in your story?
A: Simply put, I do not consider them my family; we just share the same last name. I received zero support from them when it was most needed.

Q: Did your ex-wife really break up with you in Poland?
A: Yes, she did while I was recovering, which is unheard of. She flipped and is not the same person. I continue to receive resistance from her.

Q: Did the adult stem cell procedure help?
A: I was constantly practicing walking, and this is where I saw improvement. Maybe it helped 5%, but most of the improvement came from the sweat and bruises along the way. I am glad I tried it, but unfortunately, I do not think it was helpful in my situation. It might be different for you.

Q: Did BrainPort hurt and did you notice anything?

A: There was no pain and I really liked the device; however, I did not notice any improvement. I would still recommend you try it because it might be different for you. I have seen videos and it does help people, but everyone is different; you will not know until you try.

Q: Are you fully recovered?

A: I am not fully recovered; however, I will keep practicing until I am happy with myself.

Q: Why did you write this book?

A: I wanted to help you, so you do not have to research this topic like I did, waste numerous years, and spend money where it is not needed. There was no book on this subject when I had my surgery, and this book will be your reference. I want you to recover and regain strength in your body because it can be done.

Q: How close are you to building a snowman?

A: Awfully close; I hope to try in 2020-2021.

Q: Can I contact you and will you help?

A: Yes; and yes, you may contact me at gregsiofer@iwillbewalking.com. My response might be delayed, but I will get back to you.

WHO IS GREG SIOFER?

The author of this book, Greg Siofer, knows the struggles of recovery from his own personal experience with the brain cyst operations. He felt his share of pain and helplessness, but he managed to get his life back on track. Now he wants to share his knowledge with you. This workbook of exercises is his way of helping those who need a good and reliable reference. The author's goal is to encourage others and give support to those who are just entering the battle now. Dealing with balance issues is a lot of hard work, but Greg's story is proof that you can do it, too. He likes vanilla ice cream and can be contacted by e-mail at gregsiofer@ iwillbewalking.com.

REQUEST

If you liked the information I've provided, please leave an honest review. Spread the word about this book. I want this information to reach as many people as possible to help them recover, strengthen, or just improve their balance.
Thank you,

Greg Siofer

CPSIA information can be obtained
at www.ICGtesting.com
Printed in the USA
LVHW071646131021
700337LV00004B/160